Spirituality in Health Care Contexts

of related interest

Spirituality and Mental Health Care
Rediscovering a 'Forgotten' Dimension
John Swinton
ISBN 1 85302 804 5

Spiritual Dimensions of Pastoral Care
Practical Theology in a Multidisciplinary Context
Edited by David Willows and John Swinton
Foreword by Don Browning
ISBN 1 85302 892 4

The Spiritual Dimension of Ageing
Elizabeth MacKinlay
ISBN 1 84310 008 8

Counsellors in Health Settings
Edited by Kim Etherington
Foreword by Tim Bond
ISBN 1 85302 938 6

Faith, Stories and the Experience of Black Elders
Singing the Lord's Song in a Strange Land
Anthony G. Reddie
ISBN 1 85302 993 9

Spirituality and Art Therapy
Living the Connection
Edited by Mimi Farrelly-Hansen
Foreword by Deborah Bowman
ISBN 1 85302 952 X

Psychotherapy and Spirituality
Integrating the Spiritual Dimension into Therapeutic Practice
Agneta Schreurs
Foreword by Malcolm Pines
ISBN 1 85302 975 0

Spirituality, Healing and Medicine
Return to the Silence
David Aldridge
ISBN 1 85302 554 2

Spirituality and Ageing
Edited by Albert Jewell
ISBN 1 85302 631 X

Spirituality in Health Care Contexts

Edited by Helen Orchard

Foreword by Rabbi Julia Neuberger

Jessica Kingsley Publishers
London and Philadelphia

First published in the United Kingdom in 2001 by
Jessica Kingsley Publishers Ltd
116 Pentonville Road
London N1 9JB, England
and
325 Chestnut Street,
Philadelphia, PA19106, USA

www.jkp.com

Library of Congress Cataloging in Publication Data
A CIP catalog record for this book is available from the Library of Congress

British Library Cataloguing in Publication Data
A CIP catalogue record for this book is available from the British Library

ISBN 1 85302 969 6

Printed and Bound in Great Britain by
Athenaeum Press, Gateshead, Tyne and Wear

Contents

Part Three: Cultural Contexts

Foreword

Spirituality means different things to different people – a statement of the obvious, perhaps, but one that needs unpacking for those who wish to provide spiritual care to have any understanding of what might be expected of them. Add to that the desire of many patients and users to *receive* spiritual care of some kind, without a clear definition, and it becomes apparent that this volume is long overdue and greatly to be welcomed.

For is 'spirituality' that sense of 'the other' we heard so many people describe at the time of the death of Princess Diana? Is it somewhat mawkish and sentimental, ill thought through – but 'a good thing' all the same? Does it fit with groups of young women sitting on the grass in Kensington Gardens, meditating around a candle, with masses of flowers? Or is it more to do with the angry coming to terms with impending death of the terminally ill person who recognises she has not got long to go? Or is it the mood of calm engendered by communion brought to the bedside, or the lighting of Sabbath candles? Or is it all of these things?

Helen Orchard's volume suggests it may be all of these things. Her contributors wrestle with the meaning of spirituality in a health care context, and they require auditing of the quality of spiritual care – as with any other kind of care. They worry that 'spirituality' has become a catch-all phrase for the woolly, but they argue for clarity, devotion, professionalism and, indeed, vocation.

One of the most interesting phenomena in recent years is that nurses have taken the notion of spiritual care into much of their practice and training. Part of holistic care giving, the very antithesis of the task-oriented approach, is recognising the spiritual and religious needs of patients and responding to them as far as is possible. Sometimes this can be personal, with conversation, discussion, and even shared prayer or contemplation; more often, it simply involves the recognition of a spiritual concern – and the asking of the right question at the right time. 'Would you like to see a chaplain?' or 'Can I help you find somewhere to pray?' or 'Would you like your family to come and light the Sabbath candles with you?' Even more simply, where the nurse knows little about the patient's religion, asking to be told about it often elicits a flood of information, a level of real joy at that degree of recognition, and often an idea as to what care might be most helpful and appropriate.

All in all, this volume asks many questions – of health care practitioners, of patients, of the NHS and its reductionist tendencies, and of a system where time is expensive and the care often difficult to provide. Helen Orchard and her contributors raise many tough questions and do not shy away from difficult problems. It remains for the health care community to read, inwardly digest and respond.

Rabbi Julia Neuberger
Chief Executive, The King's Fund

Acknowledgements

This book is one of the outcomes of a piece of research into hospital chaplaincy which was carried out in 1999–2000 by Lincoln Theological Institute, University of Sheffield. My thanks are due to The King's Fund, who provided the funding for the work and to Julia Neuberger for her interest in both the project and the book.

During my time at the Institute I was supported by many people with an interest in chaplaincy research. I would like especially to thank the Project Management Group – Professor David Clark, Revd Mark Cobb and Revd Dr Martyn Percy – all of whom provided significant input to the work. I am particularly grateful to Mark Cobb for his advice concerning the development of this volume.

A number of the papers collected together here were first presented at a national conference which was hosted by Lincoln Theological Institute in November 2000. I am grateful to those contributors who presented papers at the conference: Mark Cobb, Sophie Gilliat-Ray, David Lyall, Martyn Percy (for Wesley Carr), Margaret Whipp and James Woodward. I would also like to thank staff at the Institute who put a great deal of work into organising and running the conference, particularly Caroline Dicker.

Finally, my thanks again to those chaplains and other health service staff who participated in the chaplaincy research for their willingness to discuss their views and their experiences. I hope they will find this text an interesting and useful contribution.

Health Care Contexts – Spiritual Care Debates

Helen Orchard

At the inception of the NHS in 1948, a circular issued by the Ministry of Health specified that hospital authorities 'should give special attention to provide for the spiritual needs of both patients and staff' (Woodward 1998, p.90). Spiritual care has come a long way since this requirement was laid down. While it has not developed at the rate and with quite the sophistication of more technical aspects of patient care, a significant evolution has taken place nevertheless. In the last ten years in particular there has been something of a step change in the level of engagement with the spiritual care agenda by the health service. This has been the consequence of a range of factors; among them policy imperatives such as the Patient's Charter, the emergence of a holistic philosophy of health care, and the growing interest of postmodern society in what is now commonly nicknamed 'Body Mind Spirit' matters. The welcome result for the NHS has been increased debate, improved training and education and a heightened level of awareness among a whole range of health care professionals about the importance of this dimension of care. There is now an emerging plurality in the spirituality debate – the kind of plurality which inevitably attends a subject which is not owned or controlled by any one party.

This plurality is evidenced by the burgeoning number of 'Spirituality in...' books. Last year alone saw the publication of *Making Sense of Spirituality in Nursing Practice* (McSherry 2000), *Spirituality and Mental Health Care* (Swinton 2000), *Spirituality in Social Work Practice* (Abels 2000); *Psychotherapy and Spirituality* (West 2000) and *Spirituality, Healing and Medicine* (Aldridge 2000). These five represent a few of the many, but they illustrate the range of disciplines currently participating in the discussion: nursing, chaplaincy, social work, psychotherapy and psychology. To these, further partners could easily be added: medicine (Kearney 2000; Whipp 1998), pastoral theology (Jewell 1999; Willows and Swinton 2000), art and drama therapies (Farrelly-Hansen 2000; Grainger 1995) and more besides. As a contribution to the ever-growing pile, this book is under some obligation to explain its intentions to the reader. At the very least it is duty-bound to situate itself within the current field, outline its purpose and describe how it aims to fulfil it. What, then, is *Spirituality in Health Care Contexts* bringing to the table?

The book has relatively straightforward intentions. It identifies and explores three contexts in which thinking and writing about spirituality and health care are currently taking place: organisational, professional and cultural. As the titles of the texts listed above indicate, these are far from the only subjects on the spirituality agenda, but they do represent popular areas of debate at the present time. These three contexts provide the framework for the book. It is a framework which aims to promote diversity of approach but with a few deliberate constraints to hold the work together. One such constraint is the locus of attention, which has been limited to the hospital (rather than a range of health care environments) with a view to targeting the text towards the needs of a specific readership. A further intentional bias is the conscious focus on chaplaincy as the discipline under the spotlight. There is a limited amount of material written by and for this professional group and the text aims to make a particular contribution in this area. Nevertheless, an element of diversity is maintained. While the book gathers together a number of chaplaincy voices, other disciplines are also represented – nursing and medicine, theology and religious studies. Some of these contributors have long been established in this field, but others have never written for print before and the opportunity to provide a platform for some new voices was a key aim of the book. Most importantly, the perspectives of academics and practitioners sit side by side, aiming to complement each other in a manner that makes the material accessible to a wide range of readers.

Our three contexts are summarised below as a way of introducing the 'spiritual care debates' explored in each section of the book. While all of the writers bring their own unique perspective to their subject area, common strands emerge from chapters concerned with the same context. The act of drawing them together enables us to see some degree of congruence between the issues that are most exercising the contributors. Three themes are identified within each context and these are outlined briefly below, with the writers who touch on them being indicated in brackets.

Organisation as context

We begin with an attempt to focus on an area of spirituality as yet somewhat under-explored. While the literature bears witness to an interest in spirituality from both a macro (societal) and micro (individual) perspective, interest in the spiritual dimension of that unit we refer to as the organisation has been limited. In macro terms, the changing picture of faith and belief in society and the consequent impact on health care and sector ministries has been discussed (Cobb and Davie 1998; Gilliat-Ray 1999). Similarly, there has been an understandable but significant focus on the micro environment of the individual, which considers personal spirituality and ways to meet expressed need (Burnard 1988; McSherry 2000). Perhaps it is the postmodern pursuit of excessive individualism, with the consequent individualistic purchase on spirituality, which has meant that corporate aspects have received less attention. Or perhaps it is simply a question of whether it is at all possible to discuss spirituality with respect to an institution such as the NHS, or a particular health care organisation. There are those who have begun to address this question (Pattison 2000) and this section attempts to make further progress in shifting the gaze of the spiritual carer from individual to institution for a moment. A number of common themes emerge from the chapters and there is a suggestion that further exploration in this area would be fruitful.

Developing shared terminology

Despite the increasing amount of paper being generated, there often seems to be less rather than more clarity about what is meant by the term 'spirituality'. It has become a vague and diffuse notion, functioning like 'intellectual Polyfilla' which 'changes shape and content conveniently to fill the space its users devise for it' (Pattison – Chapter 2). Given that this is the situation for individual spirituality, the attempt to discuss institutional spirituality may seem even more hazardous. However, there appears to be a greater sense of general agreement in these chapters around 'what we are talking about' when referring to institutional spirituality than to its individual counterpart. Perhaps in practice it is actually easier to comprehend such a concept when considering an inanimate entity. It is, to start, far easier to make the division between religion and spirituality in this respect. A reference to an organisation's 'religion' in common parlance will generally be understood to refer to its rules and regulations, rituals and traditions. In the same way, it seems that spirituality is instinctively understood as that which constitutes an organisation's inner life or unseen workings – the forces and powers which propel it. This can be described as its group character and ethos (Lyall – Chapter 3), its ideals and 'intangible beliefs which hold all together' (Carr – Chapter 1), its values and norms (Whipp – Chapter 4). While we have perhaps not taken a quantum leap forward in terms of clarity here, we have at least started to name the domain, providing a few pegs to hang ideas on.

The importance of narrative: understanding the organisation

Perhaps the most obvious peg that emerges from considerations of institutional spirituality in this section is the importance of narrative. Stories can be used to inspect the spirituality and values within a health care organisation (Whipp, Lyall) as well as the whole edifice that is the NHS (Maltby and Pattison 1999). Narrative is a far more helpful tool than any abstract notion of spirituality because it is grounded in actuality rather than aspiration and reveals the enacted values – the 'spiritual realities' – which shape a health care organisation (Whipp). Just as personal narrative is an essential element of understanding an individual's spirituality, so too with the corporate body. This makes sense if we perceive spirituality as, in some sense, a manifestation of personality or character (Lyall). Character is inevitably disclosed by the reality of behaviour in those concrete situations that form the content of narratives.

The importance of narrative: ministering to the organisation

What does it mean to minister to an organisation's spirituality and how can this be approached? This is a concern, in one form or another, of all of the chapters in this section. The tool of theological audit can be used to develop critically the spiritual foundations on which a caring organisation is founded, aiming to make values explicit and ultimately to make change imaginable (Whipp). However, although the complexities of institutional spirituality can be analysed and to some extent understood, at the end of the day chaplains (and indeed others) can only really address them from the resources provided by their own narratives (Lyall). This fidelity to identity is viewed as an integrity crucial to the task (Pattison). Rather than becoming brokers of generic spirituality in all its forms, care givers would be more effective if they inhabited their own faith traditions more confidently, offering the experience of participating in a historically grounded, story-formed community (Pattison, Lyall).

Profession as context

The importance of a professional approach to the delivery of spiritual care has been recognised by care givers within the disciplines of both nursing and chaplaincy (McSherry 2000; Scott 2000). Nursing, which is already a significantly regulated profession, has focused on the development of training and educational programmes of varying sophistication in this area, specifying the identification of spiritual needs as one of the competencies to be achieved by all student nurses (UKCC 1986). As far as chaplaincy is concerned, while there is a perception among chaplains that the level of professionalism has increased significantly in recent years (Orchard 2000a), the professional machinery of the discipline in the UK is at an early stage. There is as yet no system of registration and a very rudimentary Code of Professional Conduct. The chapters in this section reflect the level of interest in matters professional by chaplains in particular; an interest that has been fuelled by the increased emphasis on quality, accountability and clinical governance in recent NHS policy documents (DoH 1997, 1998, 2000). Elements in the current debate are reflected by the following themes:

The professional status of spiritual care givers

While most members of the multi-disciplinary team will not be under any doubt that their occupation can be formally defined as 'a profession', chaplains are still debating the point. Although diminishing, there remains a view among some that there is an inherent conflict between a profession and a vocation and that to retain its essence, chaplaincy must remain in the latter category. The theme is explored in this section from three angles. An argument for professional status is constructed using the moral imperative of responsibility to the patient and a commitment to act for the good of others. These are considered to be the ethical grounds for professional practice, which should be promoted through the development of competencies (Cobb – Chapter 5). Another writer takes a very different starting point, using sociological approaches to understanding professions to demonstrate some of the problems in considering chaplains as professionals. The dangers of professionalisation are set out, along with the argument that retaining an element of amateurishness is essential (Woodward – Chapter 6). Similarly, the application of a postmodern critique to the health care environment reveals the impact of disciplinary power dynamics on patient care, raising questions about whether the professionalisation quest will help or hinder chaplaincy in its core task (Swift – Chapter 7). The challenge is undoubtedly to maintain a delicate balance between the notions of profession and vocation, pursuing creative and appropriate ways of developing responsible practice while maintaining the freedom afforded by a calling – more easily stated than achieved.

The identified profession of spiritual care givers

Allied to the issue of professional status for chaplaincy, and perhaps more fundamental for the service in some ways, is the question: *which* professional? Recent debates about spiritual care have suggested that it is nurses who are mapping out the terrain (Orchard 2000b) and lamented a lack of engagement by chaplains (Mitchell and Sneddon 1999). The history of the nursing profession has been used to support the primacy of their role in this area (Watson 1996), with other reasons connected with the enhancement of role and status also being suggested (Walter 1999). The question continues to generate discussion and to some extent disagreement, reflected here in several of the contributions. Nurses will clearly remain key actors in the spiritual care arena, claiming on occasion to be 'the custodian of all matters spiritual', even while they call for greater multidisciplinary collaboration in the task (McSherry – Chapter 8). Nevertheless, the dangers of blurred boundaries and widening remits are recognised: the claim by other health care disciplines to undertake spiritual care duties which are not formally attributed to them may do patients more harm than good (Cobb).

Further developing professional approaches to care

Given that the expectation of those working within the health sector is engagement in a continual process of developing their practice and improving the standard of services, one of the questions currently exercising spiritual care givers is how this can be applied to their activities. What does it mean to be a responsible and competent practitioner and how does one achieve it? Spirituality may well now be formally integrated into nurse education programmes, and basic standards exist for chaplaincy services, but what is the next stage? Four of the writers in this section grapple with this issue in different ways, encompassing the perspectives of chaplaincy and nursing. Can processes used by other health care disciplines in other scenarios be made to make sense for this challenging area of care? While a warning is sounded against appropriating scientific models for research and evidence-gathering (Swift), practical attempts are made here to develop competency frameworks (Kerry – Chapter 9), engage in ethical reflection

(Cobb) and adapt systematic nursing processes and assessment tools (McSherry). The results reveal that it is possible to mould some of these tools into a form that makes them useful for the everyday scenarios experienced by those developing and delivering care.

Culture as context

Recognising the cultural context in which spiritual and religious care are provided has become increasingly important within the health service over the last five years. This is evidenced in part by the number of texts (many of them by nurses) providing information on the cultural and religious requirements of patients from a variety of world faiths (Green 1991, Neuberger 1994, Sampson 1982). However, there has been little in the way of empirical work in this area, with Beckford and Gilliat (1996) and my own research (Orchard 2000a) being the principal examples. Contributions written specifically by leaders from minority traditions are almost non-existent, with the recent text by Sheikh and Gatrad (2000) being a notable exception. It is the scarcity of such material (compared to the glut of work on generic spirituality) which makes common themes interesting to discern and those which emerge from these chapters are outlined below.

Charting history and baselines

The lack of published material on the provision of formal spiritual care services within the health sector to minority faiths and cultures means the tasks of charting history and establishing baselines remain relevant. Basic questions – what is being provided by public funds?; by whom is it delivered?; how long has it been available? – have sketchy answers. While apocryphal tales about slow progress in advancing the multi-faith policy agenda abound in chaplaincy circles, their documentation has been limited. It is unsurprising, therefore, that outlining the history of multi-faith developments within national and local contexts is viewed as important (Lie – Chapter 14). Similarly, a snapshot of services within a specific geographical area establishes a rudimentary baseline from which a range of further empirical questions can be posed (Orchard – Chapter 11). Reviewing history and service availability are essential prerequisites for analysing current developments in the field (Gilliat-Ray – Chapter 10) and are tasks barely begun by this volume.

Discerning developing roles in minority faith groups

The developing shape of multi-faith spiritual care giving is explored here from a number of angles. A common underlying question concerns the understanding of traditional pastoral visiting practices within minority faiths. What does it mean to shift the focus from religious ritual to spiritual care for these groups of patients and indeed can such a shift be demonstrated? Practitioners address the relationship between theology and spirituality, observance of ritual and pastoral practice in Judaism (van den Bergh – Chapter 12) and Islam (Mayet – Chapter 13). Observers discuss how the Western tradition of chaplaincy is influencing the role of religious professionals in minority faiths through 'approximation' (Gilliat-Ray) and demonstrate the understanding of this phenomenon among Christian chaplains (Orchard). The impact of such shifts in role on the working of integrated chaplaincies, the wider hospital environment as well as the external cultural communities will unfold in the medium, rather than short term, as just one small facet of Britain's slow transformation into a multi-ethnic society.

Exposing the impact of inequity

A final and far from surprising theme is the lack of equitable arrangements for spiritual care for minority faiths – again, widely known but little documented. The impact on patients and carers of inequitable service provision, coupled with patchy education of health service staff, reverberates through several chapters. Structures at all levels perpetuate the status quo: from societal power structures such as Anglican patronage (Lie) and brokerage (Orchard) to institutional frameworks that regulate physical infrastructure and access to resources and remuneration (Gilliat-Ray, Lie). While the situation is slowly being addressed through gradual recruitment of minority faith 'chaplains' (Mayet, Lie, Gilliat-Ray), their absence in many organisations may have implications for the role of the Christian chaplain. An increasing emphasis on inclusivity, coupled with a little multi-faith know-how may result in the 'appropriation' of the role and responsibilities of other faiths by particular Christian denominations, broadening the scope of their remit (Orchard).

Conclusion

This introduction began by making reference to the plurality in the spirituality debate. The span and diversity of contributions in the book aim to reflect this in a manner which is creative and explorative. However, with plurality comes a latitude which does not always sit comfortably within a regulated public sector environment. The NHS is a organism that demands of its services an ability to think through its considerable complexities and to respect its need for a degree of discipline in the way care is developed and delivered. To be integrated successfully into mainstream practice, spiritual care practitioners and writers will have to attend to these needs more deliberately than has often been the case. For while there has been some excellent critical writing on spirituality from some quarters, a significant amount of the material floating about is superficial, derivative and lacking in rigour. This book aspires to make a contribution which is mindful of the need for both thoughtfulness and discipline: to discuss spirituality in health care contexts in a robust and coherent style, thereby encouraging services which are effective, equitable and better able to respond to those who call on them.

References

Abels, S. L. (2000) *Spirituality in Social Work Practice: Narratives for Professional Helping.* Denver: Love Publishing.

Aldridge, D. (2000) *Spirituality, Healing and Medicine: Return to the Silence.* London: Jessica Kingsley Publishers.

Beckford, J. A. and Gilliat, S. (1996) *The Church of England and other Faiths in a Multi Faith Society.* Warwick Working Papers in Socology 21; Warwick: University of Warwick.

Burnard, P. (1988) 'The spiritual needs of atheists and agnostics.' *Professional Nurse* December, 130–132.

Cobb, M. and Davie, G. (1998) 'Faith and belief: a sociological perspective.' In M. Cobb and V. Robshaw (eds) *The Spiritual Challenge of Health Care.* Edinburgh: Churchill Livingstone.

Department of Health (1997) *The New NHS: Modern, Dependable?* London: Department of Health.

Department of Health (1998) *A First Class Service: Quality in the New NHS.* London: Department of Health.

Department of Health (2000) *The NHS Plan: A Plan for Investment, A Plan for Reform.* London: Department of Health.

Farrelly-Hansen, M. (ed) (2000) *Spirituality and Art Therapy.* London: Jessica Kingsley Publishers.

Gilliat-Ray, S. (1999) 'Sector ministry in a sociological perspective.' In G. Legood (ed) *Chaplaincy: The Church's Sector Ministry.* London: Cassell.

Grainger, R. (1995) *The Glass of Heaven: The Faith of the Dramatherapist.* London: Jessica Kingsley Publishers.

Green, J. (1991) *Death with Dignity: Meeting the Spiritual Needs of Patients in a Multi-Cultural Society.* London: Macmillan Magazines, Nursing Times.

Jewell, A. (ed) (1999) *Spirituality and Ageing.* London: Jessica Kingsley Publishers.

Kearney, M. (2000) *A Place of Healing: Working with Suffering in Living and Dying.* Oxford: Oxford University Press.

Maltby, B. and Pattison, S. (1999) *Living Values in the NHS: Stories from the NHS's Fiftieth Year.* London: King's Fund Publishing.

McSherry, W. (2000) *Making Sense of Spirituality in Nursing Practice.* Edinburgh: Churchill Livingstone.

Mitchell, D. and Sneddon, M. (1999) 'Spiritual care and chaplaincy.' *Scottish Journal of Healthcare Chaplaincy 2,* 2, 2–6.

Neuberger, J. (1994) *Caring for People of Different Faiths.* 2nd edn; London: Mosby.

Orchard, H. (2000a) *Hospital Chaplaincy: Modern, Dependable?* Sheffield: Sheffield Academic Press.

Orchard, H. (2000b) 'Back to the bedside?' *Modern Believing 41,* 2, 2–5.

Pattison, S. (2000) 'Organisational spirituality: an exploration.' *Modern Believing 41,* 2, 12–20.

Sampson, C. (1982) *The Neglected Ethic: Religious and Cultural Factors in the Care of Patients.* Maidenhead: McGraw-Hill.

Scott, T. (2000) 'Chaplaincy – a resource of Christian presence.' *Scottish Journal of Healthcare Chaplaincy 3,* 1, 15–19.

Sheikh, A. and Gatrad A. R. (2000) *Caring for Muslim Patients.* Abingdon: Radcliffe Medical Press.

Swinton, J. (2001) *Spirituality and Mental Health Care.* London: Jessica Kingsley Publishers.

UKCC (1986) *Project 2000 – A New Preparation for Practice.* London: UKCC.

Walter, T. (1999) 'Spirituality in palliative care: opportunity or burden, prophetic vision or passing fashion.' Unpublished paper circulated by the author.

Watson, J. (1996) 'Art, caring, spirituality and humanity.' In E. Farmer (ed) *Exploring the Spiritual Dimension of Care.* Leicester: Quay.

West, W. (2000) *Psychotherapy and Spirituality.* London: SAGE Publications.

Whipp, M. (1998) 'Spirituality and the scientific mind: a dilemma for doctors.' In M. Cobb and V. Robshaw (eds) *The Spiritual Challenge of Health Care.* Edinburgh: Churchill Livingstone.

Willows, D. and Swinton, J. (eds) (2000) *Spiritual Dimensions of Pastoral Care: Practical Theology in a Multidisciplinary Context.* London: Jessica Kingsley Publishers.

Woodward J (1998) 'A Study of the Role of the Acute Health Care Chaplain in England.' Unpublished thesis of the Open University.

PART ONE

Organisational Contexts

CHAPTER 1

Spirituality and Religion
Chaplaincy in Context
Wesley Carr

In any consideration of chaplaincy the two areas of personal spirituality and the functioning of public religion, and the way that they interact, need to be addressed. In 1974 I argued that three main trends were discernible in contemporary non-theistic spirituality:

> First, this trend [towards spirituality] is away from what we might call the prophetic stream in religion or politics and towards the mystical awareness in man. Second, the character of contemporary atheism is very different from earlier forms...Alistair Kee has described the new situation as that of the 'cultural absence of God'...And thirdly, we should beware of the apparent parallels within the religious world with these attitudes from without. (Carr 1974, p.414)

Since 1974 these trends seem to have become more obvious and stronger. Yet parallel to this shift in spirituality we also have the structure of religion. This is elegantly described by David Martin in a passage that is perhaps a touch romantic but which may be destined to be one of the most quoted passages of recent English writing on religion.

> We in England live in the chill religious vapours of northern Europe, where moribund religious establishments loom over populations that mostly do not enter churches for active worship even if they entertain inchoate beliefs. Yet these establishments guard and maintain thousands of houses of God, which are markers of space and time. ... Not only are they markers and anchors, but also the only repositories of all-embracing meanings pointing beyond the immediate to the ultimate. They are the only institutions that deal in tears and concern themselves with the

breaking points of human existence. They provide frames and narratives and signs to live by, and offer persistent points of reference. ... They are – in Philip Larkin's phrase – serious places on serious earth. (Martin in Davie 1994, pp.189f)

The underlying expectation of chaplaincy

In this context, chaplaincy, a distinctive form of ministry, is exercised. Traditionally associated with hospitals and schools, it is also found in theatre and industry, as well as such specialised work as chaplaincy to farmers or tourists. Nor should we overlook the cathedrals, which today often provide chaplains with a specific ministry to visitors. All chaplaincy involves work with individuals, sometimes at considerable depth. But it usually also holds a stronger sense of addressing the institutional context than is customarily found among and expected of ministers to congregations and parish clergy. The essence of any ministry is reliability, but this is especially the case with chaplaincy. This observation gives us a clue to the context of any chaplaincy, including that in a hospital. If chaplaincy is offered, the chaplain needs to be locatable both physically – he or she has to be there – and psychologically. I offer an example from a study of industrial chaplaincy in the Diocese of Chelmsford to which I contributed some years ago. One memorable story remains with me.

On a visit to a factory on an industrial estate I found that the local industrial chaplain's presence and ministry were welcomed and valued. The factory made high technology instruments in a sterile and worker-friendly environment. We talked with people at every level – chief executive to tea boy. Most knew that there was a chaplain and who he was; many had met him. A few had made specific use of his chaplaincy, either for personal counsel or in negotiating a baptism or wedding with a local vicar. Nevertheless, nearly all valued his presence. They looked out for him each Wednesday afternoon. But when it came to articulating exactly why they valued him and what his purpose was, all fell silent or became incoherent. He was a good person; he had helped some families; the personnel department appreciated his freedom to make links with workers outside the factory. But none of these worthy reflections rang fully true, either to me or, I suspect, to the group. I sensed that there was more. Eventually, in a group discussion someone dared speak. They were glad, he said, to have a chaplain, because someone might die at work and he would know what to do. Once this was stated, there was palpable relief in the room. When asked the obvious next question – whether anyone had ever died – the answer was unsurprisingly no. But that did not matter: it was good to know the chaplain was available. Of course, this response was irrational. Such an expectation could never be met without the permanent inactive presence of a chaplain. But we found ourselves in touch with the unconscious motivations that were invested in and handled by the chaplain's role.

The dynamic interpretation

This story encapsulates a great deal about the dynamics of chaplaincy and its connection to both spirituality and religion. Like any public religious figure he or she works with people who are in a dependent mode. This description can easily be misunderstood. I am not using 'dependent' in the malign sense that is found, for example, in the phrase 'dependency culture'. Nor does it, for instance, refer to managed self-interest, contrasting being dependent with being autonomous. I use it in a technical sense derived from psychology and through that to the study of corporate and social behaviour (Reed 1978; Carr 1997; Shapiro and Carr 1991). Briefly, the argument runs that there are modes of the dynamics of human behaviour, one among which is dependence. It is basic, for it relates to the early stages of life, when the baby is dependent upon its mother for everything. When a group or institution (such as a factory, hospital or school) is in a dependent mode, it casts around for a mother figure. The members and the group as a whole invest in the belief that someone – usually an acknowledged leader, but not necessarily so – will remove the prevailing problems and relieve the stress on those who are struggling with responsibility. There are other dynamics, too. The point for this discussion is that each mode is also found not only in individuals and groups, but also in society, as these dynamics become embodied in aspects of a society (Bion 1961; Khaleelee and Miller 1985; Carr 1993). As an example, we may take another dynamic – that of fight/flight. The issue unconsciously addressed when this dynamic prevails is whether to engage in a struggle or to flee from it. In any society the armed services hold this function. We may say that they carry the fight/flight of the nation on its behalf. In other words, the military engages with hostility or threat and fights precisely so that everyone does not have to. They fight on behalf of the people and so carry 'their' fight. A society primarily locates this aspect of its life in its armed forces and, when required, mobilises it through them. Reverting to dependence, the suggestion is that religious bodies – chiefly the churches and distinctively (but not solely) where there is one, an established church – have performed this function of holding a dynamic aspect of society, and seem likely to continue to do so. As ministers go about their daily activities they are caught up, usually unwittingly, in this dimension of people's lives.

> The minister…has a great deal of hope invested in him.[1] He is asked to show dependability and reassurance, while recognizing at times that within the Church and within himself there is much uncertainty and confusion. Obvious though the point may be, it is perhaps worth restating that people turn to their Church as representing the possibility of control over events which they themselves cannot control. In particular it is asked to cope with fear of death. This means that there is inevitably an element of childlike dependency in the relationship to the Church and thus to its representatives, in that to some extent they are being asked to solve the insoluble, cure the incurable, make reality go away. Indications of this dependency are evident even among non-believers, for whom the Church symbolizes the hope of security and continuity. … For the Church the dependent posture is itself a reality that cannot be made to go away – without it the Church as an institution could scarcely exist – and so it is something to be constantly worked with. (Miller 1993, pp.106f)

This seems to me to remain true, especially when we consider public roles such as that of chaplain. Local churches are today reported to be in difficulty, although this is sometimes an assumption rather than a reality. Yet those aspects of the Church that are at the same time both marginal and central to it seem to flourish. Among these, for example, are cathedrals and greater churches. Not only are they visited as never before; they also attract congregations and significantly service local communities. There seems to be something about the anonymity of worship (as well as its reliability and style) that invites people's confidence and allows them to join, albeit temporarily, on their terms. They are points where the individual's search for some form of personal spirituality and the formal structures of religion (in this case liturgy) coincide. As Angela Tilby points out:

> …the message of usefulness is at war with the more immediate message of sheer presence and power. Cathedrals are very big, mysterious buildings. … One suspects that the understandable attempt to communicate the presence of a living community in the cathedral is not of interest to those who visit. What is much more obvious to them is the impersonality of the place. This is one Christian place of prayer where you are unlikely to be

stopped or questioned or even noticed. The messages delivered on hoardings about mission or human rights seem at odds with the buildings' containment of both good and evil in its representation of the cosmic design. Cathedrals are places of awe, not morality. (1998, p.166)

Chaplaincy: marginal but integral

What could be churchier than a bishop, dean, canons and a cathedral? These institutions are central to the church. Yet at the same time they function at its margins. They are freer than some other aspects of the church to try things. They are resourced to a surprising extent not by the church, which has regularly reduced their funding and taken away their endowments, but by local enthusiasts of various persuasions who invest in the symbolic role of 'their' cathedral.

It may at first sight seem odd to compare hospital and other chaplaincies with cathedrals. But the two themes illuminate each other. In both, the same underlying dynamic can be discerned at work, and in both, a straightforward application of the parish priest model of ministry is inappropriate. The chaplain stands in an alien and non-church environment for the Church: he or she represents it and is a focus for official questions and ecclesiastical issues. They are central figures and religion is their business. But chaplains are also marginal: they often, sometimes out of choice and sometimes because of a failure by others to understand their way of working, sit light to church structures and regard themselves on the margins of church and world. Synods and parishes are not their scene: and even the question of authority is unclear. Their milieu is often more ecumenical than most.

A specific issue is their accountability and the way that it may be divided or dispersed. Does the Anglican chaplain, for instance, report to the bishop, as licensed by him, or to a council or support group or whatever other structure is in place? There is also the other accountability to the employing trust, with a line manager ensuring adequate performance. But although the chaplain may be formally employed by the hospital, he or she may also believe that they owe a higher allegiance to God or the Church – neither of which is thought of in terms of line management. The moral dilemmas which such a position might generate are easily imagined. Here chaplains are in touch with that looser aspect of life – spirituality. They can, therefore, be called both central and marginal. They are overtly where it is publicly held that the Church ought to be – namely, 'in the world'. But they are also marginal in that their milieu is distinctive (Moody 1999). They do not customarily conform to the so-called norms of today's ministry and do not always participate in the Church's institutional life.

It is a mark of some institutions – in education and health especially – that chaplains may still be statutorily required. For example, with the advent of the National Health Service, hospitals were required to appoint chaplains. 'The chaplain was paid for his [sic] work, and was paid by money provided by Parliament. His position in the hospital was recognised and the importance of that position emphasised' (Church Information Office 1973, p.5). Changes in the Health Service both endorse and alter this expectation. Hospital trusts are required to provide for the spiritual needs of both patients and staff. But it no longer follows that this implies the appointment of a chaplain. Yet in many cases, and from whatever source chaplaincy is funded, it often seems to be a desired role. But why? In today's social context the requirement of chaplaincy is not an obvious priority. The reason, however, seems to be that he or she functions in an environment where dependence is particularly intense and dominant. This may seem strange: it is often argued that chaplaincy is carried out in secular institutions, and those that are sometimes aggressively so. In this environment, chaplains are fundamentally expected to deal with (and consequently contain) religion. Theirs is a larger concern than a matter merely of personal spirituality or the specific religious faith of individuals.

Religion is potentially a danger area for a hospital, since it is likely to pose insoluble problems for it. Like any vicar or local minister, chaplains may appear to justify their existence by doing basic 'vicar-type' things – services in the chapel, ward visits, emergency baptisms and the like. But on the basis of that performance he or she can be used by the institution to manage what is (at least unconsciously) felt to be unmanageable. Not surprisingly, therefore, many a hospital chaplain expecting to minister to the sick and dying has discovered that the ministry is more with the staff and the pressures on them than with the patients. This is not just a function of the speed of modern treatments, which keep patients in hospital for much shorter times. Many of them may never encounter the chaplain at all. But even before this modern development, it was the experience of many who work in institutions that in some sense the whole needs to be addressed and not solely individuals in need. Chaplains have, therefore, to be at home with the societal function of religion (to which they contribute) and with the personal spiritualities of those who engage with them.

The distinction is important (Carr 2000). We may think of religion as the systems of faith that are necessary if individuals are to examine their own and others' spiritualities. Spirituality, by contrast, is more private, with a greater concentration on the self and its interaction with other people and with its own inner depths. So the chaplain is often thought to be, and may behave as, marginal to the Church but an encounter with that 'centre' comes to many through his or her ministry. This marginal/central theme also relates to spirituality.

Spirituality and religion

Spirituality today is becoming a vogue theme, both within and outside the churches. There seems to be a discernible longing to recognise a spiritual dimension to existence while at the same time not turning to established religion for its articulation. For example, it was recently announced (*The Times*, 11 September 2000) that the BBC is to appoint a Head of Religion and Ethics who will preside over the present religious department. 'Mr Dyke (Director General) said the change was designed to reflect the fact that many people were now interested in spirituality without being aligned to a formal religion.' Some therapists are recognising that their work with patients may reach a boundary between therapy and spirituality that they do not feel sufficiently competent to address but which they cannot avoid or remove. Theoretical writing on this boundary is more open to reflection than has often hitherto been the case (Meissner 1984; Symington 1994). The phenomenon of the New Age, whatever precisely that is and is becoming, is an expression of longing for some sort of spirituality, often esoteric.

All this is dynamically interesting because each dimension seems to take people simultaneously into their inner world and to the boundary of their outer world. On the one hand, a person's spirituality is eclectically their own. This is true of everyone, whether a member of a church or synagogue or any person indulging their own wishes. It is always salutary to clergy and ministers to be reminded that they do not know what their congregation believes, whatever they may be saying, singing or hearing. On the other hand, spirituality also pushes people to the boundaries of their self-awareness and existence, and is rarely solitary: there seems to be almost a compulsion to make links with like-minded people.

The two issues of spirituality and religion focus and unite in the person of the chaplain. He or she represents religion and it is impossible to do that without being religiously and denominationally specific. But the chaplain will also be called upon to affirm aspects of the spirituality, not just of the patients but often that of the institution too.

This recent encounter will serve to illustrate the point. At a formal dinner I met a senior person in national life who would be accounted by most people as among the great and the good. She had been the chairperson of a Regional Health Authority. She was also on the council of a new university. She talked about the church (to which she actively belonged) and about chaplaincy to the university. It was an interesting and stimulating conversation. But she came even more alive later in the evening when for some reason the question of angels came up. She suddenly announced that she had angels everywhere: she meant (although the statement was not unambiguous) images and pictures of angels. These reinforced her strong belief in angelic presence and effectiveness in guiding people through life – at least for her. The easy slide in such an establishment figure from the need for properly functioning structural religion into personal belief was both remarkable and characteristic of our age. She did not appear to sense any disjunction between the two. But the episode was qualitatively different from what I have experienced throughout most of my ministry. The topic of religion, though customarily avoided at polite dinner tables, might have been risked with a dean. The intimacies of personal belief, however, (especially in something as idiosyncratic as angels) would have been kept private.

This story further illustrates the location of the chaplain (although in this instance it was a dean) at both the centre and the margins. I was engaged in this conversation as representing the centre, a senior representative of the Church and its organisational effectiveness (or otherwise) in addressing the religious questions of a number of institutions. But I was simultaneously involved in the margins, as someone who was expected to know about the esoteric question of angels – and, what is more, be understanding and sympathetic to this person's specific belief. I could, of course, argue about the Church amicably and authoritatively. So could my companion, who could speak from her lay experience in a parish and university. But the presented personal belief was felt to be and was treated as inviolable and could not be challenged.

This vignette raises interesting issues about the boundary between religion and spirituality, which is where the chaplain works. For example, the discussion was based on the assumption that religion was public, organisational and clearly definable in terms of the roles of the speaker (church person) and me (authorised minister). But there were also boundary issues between the ways in which that religion had held for generations mention of angels. Without that tradition she would not have known about angels, and her intense personal development of almost a private angelology in her own self-regarding spirituality could not have occurred. I – and in similar circumstances any chaplain would, too – oscillated between the public and the private domains. The role, therefore, was determined by the data. Religious and spiritual life, in spite of the oft-made assumption today that spirituality can sit light to formal religion, are both central and marginal.

Aspects of the chaplain's role

From this brief discussion four aspects of the chaplain's role in this context can be distilled. All may not apply to all, but somewhere they are around most ministries in institutions. They are not in any ranked order of importance

Manager

Sometimes the chaplain manages territory (a chapel) and sometimes ritual (worship and rites of passage). But there is always something in an institution's life that is felt to be unmanageable and for which people may look to the chaplain for management. Worship is an obvious example. Chapel worship or services on wards used to be a substitute for worship for those who were temporarily resident in the new 'parish' of the hospital. With shorter patient stays and staff shift work, there is rarely a firm base for a worshipping congregation. Yet it is fascinating to observe that for most chaplains some liturgical activity remains part of their ministry. The service is not just for those few who attend: it is expected of a 'proper' chaplain and represents a way of identifying his or her basic role, which is religious. Once that is established, the chaplain can engage in that informal exploration of thanksgiving or despair which goes on throughout life but which often surfaces *in extremis* in hospital. This is also more intensely true of ministry in a hospice, where the congregational aspect to public worship is stronger. There is also likely to be some connection between the inner life of the individual – the private spirituality and the recognition of sufficient religious structure – and the role of the chaplain in both areas.

Arbiter

Religion carries intense, however diffuse, feelings in a society. This function is likely to be even more acute in specific settings, such as a hospital, college or university. There are gods everywhere. The pervasiveness and persistence of religion may surprise a modern, secular institution. From time to time, the multi-religious nature of modern plural society means that the institution may need a perspective on specific religions.

Although a controversial stance, I judge that it is no answer simply to appoint large, multi-faith chaplaincy teams. For in reality there is not that supply of men and women available and when finance again bites, they are vulnerable to cost–benefit questions. And second, the managers of the institution need to be able to acquire basic information about religious custom, belief and practice before handling whatever issue arises. Here a chaplain's authority gives him or her a primary function as representative of religion in general with the skills, like that of any minister, of theology and learning.

Facilitator

Because the chaplain usually sits structurally loose to the system, he or she may occupy almost any place. The model is illustrated by chaplaincy in the Royal Navy. There the chaplain is regarded as holding the rank of the person to whom he is speaking. People often look in curious places for sanctions by which they may be let-be and encouraged. In this role the chaplain may be serving the institution (religion) while addressing someone's most personal beliefs (spirituality).

Interpreter

Every day and everywhere, people are looking for ways to interpret their fragments of life experience within the larger whole, whatever that may be at any moment. For patients in hospital, even those with the most bravura, ultimate issues of life and its quality and inevitably death are faced. The staff face similar pressures. To contain these and make them manageable, structures are developed both deliberately and unconsciously (Menzies 1967). While the chaplain cannot claim a role here, it is possible that, because of the ambiguous position (between centre and margin, between religion and spirituality, between institutional role and person) that he or she occupies, the chaplain can be used to interpret what may be happening to people. The chaplain's own perspective is itself always being enlarged. He or she, therefore, may be in a privileged position to be used as an interpreter for the institution from an involved but separate stance.

'Spirituality of the institution'

There remains one further area to be addressed. Chaplains are appointed by an institution to work within it. Talking with chaplains, too, they will often reflect on their value to the institution, usually in terms of appreciation. The hospital chaplain, as we have noted, does not just meet patients and administer rites. However, those who work in the hospital become increasingly his or her clients. As stress in the system becomes more acute, and ethical questions become more immediate, so the chaplain – if good at the job – is turned to for pastoral care. This is a big subject. When, however, we emphasise the aspect of 'institution', ideals become important. The reason for this is that 'institution' is a shared concept. The participants generate a series of 'institutions-in-the-mind' with which they negotiate with one another what the body is and what they are about. This approach emphasises motivation arising from belief and a sense that values are affirmed. And by values we may mean both general ideals as well as specific values – those things to which priority has currently to be given and for which all not only do work but more importantly also wish to work. Jaques and Clement (1991) remark: 'It is our values that move us, bind us together, push us apart, and generally make the world go round' (p.73).

This area may be described as 'the spirituality of the institution' – that intangible but necessary set of engaged beliefs that hold all, whatever their specific roles, together (Carr 1999). The link between personal and institutional spirituality may in fact be the most critical area for the contemporary chaplain. While not there specifically to boost morale or encourage the workers, he or she is part of the system but not wholly of it. Chaplains are available with the offer of pastoral care and in many cases, when the privilege has been earned through faithful ministry, they may contribute to ethical and (we may say) spiritual exploration, both personal and institutional.

Note

1. In 1973 when this note was written, women had not been ordained as priests in the Church of England, although some were deaconesses or licensed workers. Chaplaincy was one of the major opportunities open to them then. Other churches, of courses, had women ministers.

References

Bion, W. R. (1961) *Experiences in Groups and Other Papers.* London: Tavistock Publications.

Carr, A. W. (1974) 'Contemporary non-theistic spirituality.' *Theology 77,* 650, 412–417.

Carr, A. W. (1993) 'Some consequences of conceiving society as a large group.' *Group: The Journal of the Eastern Group Psychotherapy Society 17,* 4, 235–244.

Carr, A. W. (1997) *Handbook of Pastoral Studies.* London: SPCK.

Carr, A. W. (1999) 'Can we speak of the "Spirituality of Institutions"?' In J. Coble and C. Elliott (eds) *The Hidden Spirit: Discovering the Spirituality of Institutions.* Matthews NC: Christian Ministry Resources.

Carr, A. W. (2000) 'Some reflections on spirituality, religion and mental health.' *Mental Health, Religion and Culture 3,* 1, 2–12.

Church Information Office (1973) *The Hospital Chaplain – A Report of the Working Party Appointed by the Joint Committee.* London: Church Information Office.

Davie, G. (1994) *Religion in Britain since 1945. Believing without Belonging.* Oxford: Blackwell.

Jaques, E. and Clement, S. (1991) *Executive Leadership: A Practical Guide to Managing Complexity.* Oxford: Blackwell.

Khaleelee, O. and Miller, E. J. (1985) 'Beyond the small group: society as an intelligible field of study.' In M. Pines (ed) *Bion and Group Psychotherapy.* London: Routledge and Kegan Paul.

Meissner, W. W. (1984) *Psychoanalysis and Religious Experience.* New Haven: Yale University Press.

Menzies, I. E. P. (1967) 'A case-study in the functioning of social systems as a defense against anxiety.' *Human Relations 13,* 95–121.

Miller, E. J. (1993) *From Dependency to Autonomy. Studies in Organisation and Change.* London: Free Association Books.

Moody, C. (1999) 'Spirituality and sector ministry.' In G. Legood (ed) *Chaplaincy: The Church's Sector Ministries.* London: Cassell.

Reed, B. D. (1978) *The Dynamics of Religion: Process and Movement in Christian Churches.* London: Darton, Longman and Todd.

Shapiro, E. R. and Carr, A. W. (1991) *Lost in Familiar Places. Making New Connections between the Individual and Society.* New Haven and London: Yale University Press.

Symington, N. (1994) *Emotion and Spirit. Questioning the Claims of Psychoanalysis and Religion.* London: Cassell.

Tilby, A. (1998) 'The Sacred Grove. Cathedrals and Cosmic Religion.' In S. Platten and C. Lewis (eds) *Flagships of the Spirit. Cathedrals in Society.* London: Darton, Longman and Todd.

CHAPTER 2

Dumbing Down the Spirit

Stephen Pattison

Strictly speaking, the only essential qualification that Christian chaplains must possess for working in health care is their ordination, with, by, and through the power of the Holy Spirit (Woodward 1999). However, in a world in which religions in general and Christianity in particular have become something of an embarrassing anachronistic irrelevance, it is often held that, while there is a spiritual aspect to life and everyone has spiritual needs, only some people express these needs in terms of religion (Speck 1988).

So what are chaplains, products, representatives, even icons, of a specific tradition supposed to do with their religious roots and perceptions? Are they to leave their origins, rituals, teachings and traditions behind? Should they regard them as an optional resource for those who can make use of 'that kind of thing' while trying to act as spiritual guides and mentors for all, religious or not? Or do they need to find a new, lively accommodation with the religious traditions that have shaped them and which have provided pathways to God?

The underlying question here is, should specifically theistic religion, with all that that implies in terms of belief, knowledge and practice, have a central place within health care provision today? Or is it time that particular religious groups and their representatives, including chaplains, were removed from their publicly-funded positions to the margins of private life and personal choice so that a more universally acceptable kind of meaning system encompassed by a general term such as 'spirituality' can take its place? Correlatively, is it appropriate that representatives of particular religious traditions should become much more closely identified with their own specific religious roots? This might enable them to enrich the tapestry of religious and spiritual discourse with their own insights and wisdom rather than having to present a sanitised, homogenised, generalised spiritual concern.

If 'spirituality' in general terms is more desirable than religion, it is unclear what part representatives of religious communities should play in delivering 'spiritual care'. Indeed, it is precisely because of their specifically religious origins and training that chaplains as representatives of particular religious views and communities may be the last people suitable for facilitating or providing 'spiritual care' in the generic, secularised sense that seems now to be prevalent across a variety of professions (Cobb and Robshaw 1998; McSherry and Draper 1997; Ross 1995). It could be argued that if the promotion of generic, religiously neutral spiritual care is the ideal in health care, then nurses, existential counsellors, or philosophers might be better suited to providing care and assistance than chaplains.

While it may be in the interests of short-term pragmatic expediency for chaplains to sit light to their religious origins in the name of attending to matters of spirituality and spiritual care more broadly, this may not be in their own or others' long-term interests. For generalised 'spirituality', while it may be more acceptable than religion, has many aspects which are inimical to, and very different from, those that characterise historic religious traditions by which generations of believers have lived and died. Furthermore, the gradual subordination of religious commitment and practice to a more generalised spiritual quest is liable to weaken the capacity of religious traditions usefully to contribute to such a quest in the long term. I find it difficult to see much future or lasting value for floating spiritualities divorced from communities of practice and discourse where they have been tested and refined over centuries.

The casualty of substituting 'spiritual care' for religious care may be that much wisdom and insight, welcome or unwelcome, is lost in the interests of providing bespoke metaphysical marshmallow that is non-specific, unlocated, thin, uncritical, dull and un-nutritious. Pastoral care which transmutes into generic spiritual care may become a case of the bland leading the bland.

I want to argue here that religion, specifically Christian religion, is a substantive tradition that must be addressed and lived with rather than subordinated within chaplaincy. Furthermore, I believe that the Christian tradition of Spirit and spirituality, like that of many other historic religions, has little to do with contemporary notions of 'spirituality'. This tradition, rooted in theism, is distinctive, specific, embarrassing and challenging when compared to vague nostrums of spirituality and spiritual care which may owe more to philosophy than to religion. This means that it has all the advantages and disadvantages of an ambivalent, inhabited and living historic tradition, both radical and conservative, that make spirituality worth attending to in the first place. I suggest that chaplains need to re-evaluate their relationship with and responsibility for their own particular spiritual tradition rather than uncritically attempting to become generic facilitators or brokers of spirituality in all its manifestations from Wicca to Buddhism.

One way of developing the points made above is to bring out the distinction made briefly above that spirituality, in the generic sense that is often used around health care, has little to do with Christian spirituality. To establish this, I will now look more carefully at the tradition of Christian spirituality. I will then examine some of the main characteristics of generic spirituality and spiritual need.

Spirit and spirituality in the Christian tradition

The Christian spiritual tradition has been pluriform and multi-vocal. However, it should be uncontroversial to suggest that it has its roots and much of its ongoing sustenance in biblical insights into the nature of Spirit and spirituality. After centuries of established churches and conventional religion, often closely allied to dominant social institutions and ideologies, it can easily be forgotten that the roots of this religion are in charismatic theism (Weber 1963). So what can be learned about the nature of Spirit and spirituality from Christian biblical pneumatology?

In the first place, the Spirit is divine and transcendent. While it touches human life and can be identified with it (e.g. in terms like 'human spirit') as its creator and quickener, it is independent and goes beyond human knowledge and experience (cf Gen. 1:2; Ps.18:15). To encounter the Spirit is to encounter the divine and holy – with all the fear and awe that that suggests.

Second, the Spirit is active – it takes initiatives and it is not just to be found passively waiting to be discovered by mystics or philosophers somewhere inside the human psyche. To be inspired or inspirited is to encounter divine otherness that comes from outside the human realm:

> 'Spirit' is the word used from the earliest traditions behind the OT to denote the mysterious invisible power of God, manifested in the wind…, in the breath of life…and in the ecstatic power of charismatic leader and prophet. (Dunn 1983, p.357. Cf Lindblom 1962; Witherington 2000)

Furthermore, this experience is likely to be a demand for action and change, a summons to obedience to God's will, not an affirmation of the status quo. It should be remembered here that Jesus' first experience of the Spirit described in Mark 1:12 was the disturbing, alienating one of being thrown out into the desert, not a warm inner glow of happiness and self-realisation. The work of the Spirit draws people into the passion and resurrection of Jesus Christ. This is daunting and dangerous.

Third, the effects of the Spirit's work are not wholly or even mainly confined to individuals. In Pauline theology, the work of the Spirit is to build up the whole people of God (cf I Cor. 12:4ff). Furthermore, the Spirit is concerned with corporate and political reality as much as it is with individuals, a fact to which the ministry of the prophets bears clear witness (Lindblom 1962).

Fourth, the Spirit's work is bound up with the whole of material reality and it can effect changes such as healings within it (Gen. 1:2; cf Wink 1984). The Holy Spirit is not a ghost in the sense of being a disembodied wraith. There is a spiritual aspect to every part of creation, including the human creation. It is not for nothing that the Spirit's work is associated with basic elements such as wind and fire (Acts 2:1ff).

Fifth, the Spirit is associated with real power to change, bend and burn that which is contrary to the will and purposes of God. It literally inspires people and transforms them in unpredictable ways. While the 'voice' of the Spirit may sometimes be low and still, the primary characteristic of Spirit is that of divine power that cannot be resisted.

Finally, the Spirit is not biddable or amenable to human manipulation. The Spirit blows where it wills, accomplishing the will and purposes of God (cf Jn. 3:8). It is not a spiritual 'resource' like electricity that can be channelled and turned on and off according to human whim. The Spirit is unpredictable, as many who have wanted to control it have found. It refuses to inspire or heal on command and works in places where it has no business to be. It is in the light of these characteristics that it is possible to understand that 'To think deeply about the Holy Spirit is a bewildering, tearing exercise, for whatever he [sic] touches he turns it inside out' (Taylor 1972, p.177).

The view of Spirit as divine, independent, active, demanding, social, materially related, powerful and unbiddable in the interests of revealing God's will and perfecting creation is central to a biblically informed Christian spirituality. This charismatic theistic tradition is not an easy one to assimilate into the modern world. Aspects of it are ambivalent, even embarrassing and dangerous. So, for example, the notion of signs, healings and wonders accomplished by forces that are unbiddable and outwith human control is deeply suspect within the context of contemporary health care with its emphasis upon scientific rationality and managed predictability (Pattison 2000a).

It is not surprising, then, that Christian chaplains are not particularly keen to promote knowledge of their tradition. They may be tempted to opt in to a more generalised and less specific language about spirituality that is more sanitised and acceptable in the modern world. This dumbing down of the heart of Christian discipleship and spirituality may have much to be said for it in terms of attaining acceptance and inclusion. However, there are losses as well as gains here. This becomes apparent when one looks at the rather emaciated, limited and vague notions of 'spirituality' that presently obtain in the health care arena generally.

'Spirituality' in health care

Spirituality has become a very important category for understanding the condition of individual patients or users within health care today. The impetus to identify and attend seriously to this dimension of existence received a powerful boost from the Patient's Charter (DoH 1991). This was taken to suggest that users were entitled to have their spiritual as well as their other needs met within health services. The Charter did not provide a definition of 'spiritual needs', but their inclusion has helped to fuel a quest to define and meet such needs subsequently. Many professional groups, especially nurses and chaplains, have become engaged in the quest to identify and meet spiritual needs effectively as can be seen from contributions to volumes like Cobb and Robshaw's *The Spiritual Challenge of Health Care* (1998).

This book reveals that notions of 'spirituality' that are presently in play are diffuse, vague and contradictory. 'Spirituality' seems to function like intellectual Polyfilla, changing shape and content conveniently to fill the space its users devise for it. Having mostly departed from the theories and practices of religion, theorists and practitioners of spirituality are muddled about what actually constitutes their subject matter.

Some contributors to the book see spirituality as having a lot to do with formal faith and religion – hence, presumably, the appropriateness of involving clergy in it. Many want to preserve some kind of non-specified notion of transcendence while carefully excluding the divine as a necessary part of that transcendent dimension. Others see spirituality as having to do with the realm of ethics and morals embodied in notions like respect. A number of writers conceive of spirituality as a kind of humanistic limit concept whereby that which cannot easily be expressed but which is felt to be a kind of unthought known in human existence is rendered non-specifically visible and significant. At the other end of the scale, there are those who want quickly to reduce the 'spiritual' to some features of empirically observable behaviour and existence that can clearly be specified and thus directly addressed, for example by the provision of specific spiritual care. Over against these writers are those who want to use spirituality as a kind of protest against reductionism and exclusion of important aspects of human existence that cannot easily be described and discussed in other terms.

There are, however, a number of assumptions that unite most of the book's contributors. First, spirituality is an unequivocally 'good thing'. It is universally valid and valued. Everyone does and should have 'it', and because they do, they should have their spiritual needs, however defined, met. There appears to be no such thing as a dubious spirituality, a harmful spirituality, or one that should not be indulged. (Compare Wakefield's pertinent observation that Hitler had a powerful spirituality but it was not a beneficial one (1983, p.362).)

Second, there seems to be some consensus on the idea that spirituality and spiritual needs can be identified, measured and met. Thus the realm of the spiritual is commodified and reduced to predictable service rather than a category of the unknown and unknowable.

Third, it seems largely to be agreed that spirituality is an individual matter that has mostly to do with the well-being of persons, not groups or communities. Individualism in focus here mirrors the individualism of health and social care generally.

Fourth, there is no kind of well-founded and -tried community, practice or discipline that surrounds and sustains the seeker after spiritual reassurance or wisdom. It is up to the individual to find her own way to transcendence and connection, preferably quickly so existential angst can be avoided in the context of illness.

Fifth, the assumption seems to be that since health care is basically the province of professionals, there must be some professionals around who can make a career out of expertly diagnosing and meeting spiritual needs. Thus it is a matter of identifying professional appropriateness and expertise for dealing with spirituality, not a matter of acknowledging that spirituality might be beyond the competence and range of particular professional groups.

Finally, although this is not explicitly acknowledged, spirituality seems to extend no further than some kind of Stoic accommodation with the individual's life, reality and beliefs. No metaphysics are required here. Spirituality is just how you get on with accepting the inevitable, adjusting to it, and wresting meaning from it (cf Karp 1996).

This combination of features suggests, contra Markham (1998), that contemporary thinking about spirituality is much closer to the thought and practice of certain kinds of philosophy, particularly the atheistic therapeutic philosophies such as Stoicism and Epicureanism, than it is to religion as it has mostly been understood (Nussbaum 1994). It has, as far as I can see, almost no relationship to theistic religion at all. Furthermore, it cannot have such a relationship if it is to be acceptable in the secularised public market place of health care amongst people of all faiths and none.

In the next part of this chapter I want to point out some of the real advantages of maintaining a religiously distinctive and critical standpoint in health care chaplaincy and spirituality rather than seeking to become all things to all people in the name of a vague kind of spiritual relevance that may ultimately prove to be ephemeral and illusory. Maintaining religious identity and discipline might be one of the gifts that chaplains can offer to health care, even if this is not so immediately acceptable and gratifying as unlocated spirituality.

The value of Christian religion in the spiritual context

There is a considerable difference between Christian spirituality and religion, based on historic and communally founded theistic belief in an active God who evokes response through the Holy Spirit, and the contemporary quest for generic spirituality in health care. It is entirely understandable, even evangelically responsible, for Christian chaplains to wish to be universally helpful in the area of spiritual care. However, I want to argue that they might more usefully situate themselves as religious functionaries within a rich and distinctive religious tradition. It is my belief that the effective abandonment of a particular charismatic theistic spirituality in favour of generic consumer 'spirituality' may lead to the long-term impoverishment of all concerned.

Resisting the fall into spiritual Esperanto

Surveying the many fundamentally different discourses about ethics in the postmodern world, Stout (1988) observes that there is a temptation to try to develop a lowest common denominator moral language that all participants can 'speak' and agree upon – a kind of moral Esperanto. However, the problem with Esperanto is that it belongs to all communities and to none. Speakers of Spanish or English may have difficulty in understanding each other and have to make considerable efforts to communicate. However, the languages that they speak are grounded in particular communities and have important utterances written and spoken in them. Nobody, on the other hand, has yet written anything of importance in Esperanto. Few people bother to learn this 'ideal' language that promises to solve all the world's communication problems. Thus it remains essentially trivial and unimportant.

There is perhaps a similar difficulty with the pursuit of generic spirituality that embraces all people. While none are excluded, such a sterile, non-located area of concern may have little of value and substance to offer, least of all those who face problems of life and death. According to Stout, the answer to pluralism and inclusiveness in morality is not to eliminate distinctive communities and languages and to sink all differences. Rather, people should take the trouble to learn each other's languages and cultures. This is a more interesting and profitable exercise than trying to identify lowest common denominators or to globalise common ways of thinking, speaking and acting. Boundaries are not best dealt with by eliminating or ignoring them. Rather, taking them seriously can be a source of insight and growth for all concerned.

If this kind of thinking is applied in the arena of spiritual care, what may be most needed is not a concern for generic lowest common denominator eclectic spirituality with no insiders or outsiders (and, by implication, no distinctive communities of belief and practice who provide both insights and challenges). Rather, confident inhabitants of particular faith traditions who are prepared to dialogue honestly with others are required. In this context, the duty of Christian chaplains might be to be competent witnesses and exponents of their own faith traditions and communities, not facilitators for the spiritualities of the world.

The need for identity and integrity – an end to spiritual brokerage

Due to the muddled usage of the term 'spirituality', and the fact that in the West this has often been associated directly with the Christian tradition, it is not surprising that Christian chaplains have allowed themselves to become brokers of 'spirituality' generally and not just representatives of their own tradition (Orchard 2000). There is much to be commended in this open-minded, concerned attitude for people of all faiths and none. It is a great advance on tribalism, exclusivism, and xenophobia. However, there is much that may be glossed over and lost here. In particular, chaplains may be tempted to downplay the importance of their own tradition and identity within that tradition in the interests of being universally accepting and acceptable. In the long term, this can only weaken their value as speakers of a particular language and representatives of a particular religious community and tradition.

The advantages of such a tradition are that it brings to situations of life and death real wisdom and integrity of character and belief. While this may appal some, and be unhelpful to others, particular religious traditions and practices that have emerged from human experience over millennia should not be discarded unthinkingly, particularly by those who appear to be their most prominent representatives in health care settings. A faithful spiritual journey within any religious tradition is likely to be demanding, involving personal and communal conflict and difficulty. However, the outworking of that journey is likely to be of value to those both inside and outside that tradition. If chaplains and other religious representative persons abandon the value of their own religious traditions, what do they really have to offer those who are spiritually needy and lost? And if Christian chaplains insist on seeing themselves as brokers for all religious traditions and none in the provision of spiritual care, what chance is there that health care institutions and users of different faiths and none can really gain something of lasting value from the Christian or any other tradition?

At stake here is the issue of religious identity and integrity. As long as Christian chaplains see themselves as generic brokers of spiritual care of all kinds, they are in danger of forsaking what they most distinctively and usefully have to offer; their lived experience of dwelling within a historic religious tradition by which people over centuries have lived and died. Furthermore, as 'universal' spiritual brokers, they may risk distorting and misrepresenting the faith traditions of others who should be allowed to speak and minister for themselves.

The implication of this argument is that representatives of Christianity should be seen as such, not as managers or brokers of generic spiritual care. And working alongside such representatives, there should be those of other faiths and none who should be allowed to communicate their own insights and practices in their own way. It is only when we stop being universal figures, as 'men' were thought to be in sexist language, that both Christian and other faith inhabitants will be able to find and fully express their own religious identities.

I suspect that underlying the apparent liberal universalism of 'spiritual' as opposed to pastoral care lies a good deal of uncritical assumption that Christian (especially, perhaps, Anglican) ministers can really be all things to all people. Furthermore, all religions and spiritualities are valid and lead to the same place, so everyone can be accommodated within the supermarket of spiritual need. This kind of thinking is criticised in many types of inter-religious dialogue. It often leads to an unwitting imperialism and 'baptism' of others' beliefs and practices. This is deeply unacceptable to those others (D'Costa 1986). To be respectful to others as a Christian chaplain may most appropriately involve being deeply Christian in one's own ideas and practices, not accommodating others within some kind of web of 'spiritual care' that they have not consented to inhabit.

The need for theological critique and 'prophecy'

Generic spiritual care provision within health care is muddled and contested. Spirituality is taken to be a universal personal need that must be met within health care. A broad, vaguely philosophical, personal quest for meaning, value, worth etc. may be perfectly valid in its own terms. However, it has little or nothing to do with Western religious traditions generally, or the Christian religious tradition in particular.

Indeed, the Christian spiritual tradition can be taken to be in many ways highly critical of many of the assumptions upon which contemporary generic 'spirituality' rests. If chaplains can access and retain aspects of their theological and spiritual tradition there is much insight of a usefully critical nature which they might offer to enrich the rather vacuous discussion about spiritual care. While some of this might be controversial, problematic, or even offensive, judiciously offered religious and theological 'fragments' (Forrester 1997) may provide some kind of time-tried grit for a discourse that otherwise risks trivialisation. Thus it may be possible to transcend the worthy dullness of spiritual Esperanto and the sickly dangers of metaphysical marshmallow. As the lives of the holy ones in religious traditions show, such grit can in fact produce pearls.

Where generic spirituality is not theistic, Christian spirituality is. While generic spirituality is seen as a quest for meaning for its own sake, Christian spirituality is essentially a response to the action of a transcendent God incarnate in Jesus Christ. The Spirit is given to accomplish God's will on earth, a universal commission. It is not a controllable, comprehensible commodity that can be distributed according to human priorities and needs. The Spirit to which Christians respond is gracious and beneficent but not biddable. Furthermore, it is not predictable or controllable – it is literally inspiring (as opposed to much generic spirituality which might be characterised as ex-spiring). The Spirit can be destructive and challenging rather than comforting. While it may certainly comfort the afflicted, it also afflicts the comfortable, demanding obedience and change.

The scope of the Spirit's concern and the limit of Christian spirituality is the whole of bodily life and creation, not the mind or soul of the person. While the individual may be important within Christian charismatic spirituality, the whole thrust of Christian spirituality is towards creating and building up communities of faith. Christian spirituality encompasses all material, social and political realities (Pattison 2000b). So an important part of its pursuit includes the quest for social and political justice and change (Sheldrake 1987). The place where people learn about and co-operate with the Spirit, i.e. engage in spirituality, is the community of the faithful, commissioned by God to engage in the work of salvation. So this spirituality is outward-looking, altruistic and socially concerned. It makes substantial moral demands upon adherents who are supposed to manifest the gifts of the Spirit, not just to feel that life has meaning and value.

The implication of this is that the place where the Spirit is discerned is within the worshipping community, its scriptures, rituals and practices of prayer, not in individual introspection. Communal belonging and identity is challenging. However, the Spirit makes it possible for those open to its promptings to transcend themselves and discover love and belonging. Thus the disciplines of prayer, worship and work provide a clear way of working with and for God that is lacking in the generic quest to meet spiritual needs which tends to be individualistic, introspective, personal and quietistic.

It is this fiery, transcendent and, in some ways, difficult charismatic spiritual tradition to which Christian chaplains are heirs. However, it has been effectively dumbed down by contemporary Christians, keen to be all things to all people. If discriminatingly used and understood, it might provide considerable fruitful material for thinking with and against, both within and outside the Christian community. For example, becoming more clear about the theologies underlying Christian spirituality might help make other stakeholders within the world of spiritual care a bit clearer about their own teleologies and anthropologies, whether or not they find the Christian ones acceptable (Pattison 1997).

Distinctively Christian religious spirituality should not be casually downplayed or discarded. It may figure a larger, more interesting and better developed, if more problematic, understanding of spirituality and how it might be pursued than many of the anaemic 'available on prescription' generic spiritualities that are presently washing around the NHS. Above all, perhaps, it provides lived performances of spirituality which can be examined, understood, criticised and imitated rather than vague promises or Stoic nostrums. While the latter may not be worthless, they have not yet decisively demonstrated their capacity to nourish and inspire body, mind and spirit in this secular age. For Christians, finding personal meaning and individual acceptance is not enough. The Christian life is about praise, worship and work in community with an active loving God, not just about passive endurance in an empty universe (Hardy and Ford 1984). Perhaps it is time that chaplains were more willing to remind themselves and others of this as their distinctive contribution to the Babel surrounding 'spirituality' in health care and elsewhere.

Conclusion

None of what I have written here should be construed as a manifesto for retreat on the part of Christian chaplains or others into exclusivism, religiosity, nostalgia, or triumphalist evangelisation within the sphere of health care. My purpose here has been to suggest that chaplains who come from a distinctive and valuable religious tradition should think more carefully about what it is that they can bring into the fragmented world of generic spirituality. Given the dominance of institutional Christianity in Britain in the past, it is perhaps appropriate that Christian representatives should not push their own tradition aggressively. However, it is getting to a point where people have only the haziest idea of what that tradition is and what it might have to offer by way of wisdom and life-enhancing disciplines.

The churches in general and chaplains in particular perhaps need to think harder about the use that they can appropriately, creatively and non-oppressively make of their own native theologies and practices within the health care arena. It is my belief that they will not serve users, health care institutions, or the future of chaplaincy best by dumbing down the Spirit and forgetting their own tradition in the interests of promoting generic 'spiritual care'. Indeed, if they do not engage more directly with that tradition, there is a real danger that it will be diminished and die so that a major source of insight and challenge will be denied to generations yet to come.

References

Cobb, M. and Robshaw, V. (eds) (1998) *The Spiritual Challenge of Health Care.* Edinburgh: Churchill Livingstone.

D'Costa, G. (1986) *Theology and Religious Pluralism.* Oxford: Blackwell.

Department of Health (1991) *The Patient's Charter.* London: HMSO.

Dunn, J. (1983) 'Holy Spirit.' In G. Wakefield (ed) *A Dictionary of Christian Spirituality.* London: SCM Press.

Forrester, D. (1997) *Christian Justice and Social Policy.* Cambridge: Cambridge University Press.

Hardy, D. and Ford, D. (1984) *Jubilate: Theology in Praise.* London: Darton, Longman and Todd.

Karp, D. (1996) *Speaking of Sadness.* Oxford: Oxford University Press.

Lindblom, J. (1962) *Prophecy in Ancient Israel.* Oxford: Blackwell.

Markham, Ian (1998). 'Spirituality and the world faiths.' In M. Cobb and V. Robshaw (eds) *The Spiritual Challenge of Health Care.* Edinburgh: Churchill Livingstone.

McSherry, W. and Draper, P. (1997) 'The spiritual dimension: why the absence within nursing curricula?' *Nurse Education Today 17,* 413–417.

Nussbaum, M. (1994) *The Therapy of Desire.* Princeton: Princeton University Press.

Orchard, H. (2000) *Hospital Chaplaincy: Modern, Dependable?* Sheffield: Sheffield Academic Press.

Pattison, S. (1997) *The Faith of the Managers.* London: Cassell.

Pattison, S. (2000a) 'Some objections to aims and objectives.' In G. Evans and M. Percy (eds) *Managing the Church?* Sheffield: Sheffield Academic Press.

Pattison, S. (2000b) 'Organisational spirituality: an exploration.' *Modern Believing 41,* 2, 12–20.

Ross, L. (1995) 'The spiritual dimension: its importance to patients' health, well-being and quality of life and its implications for nursing practice.' *International Journal of Nursing Studies 32,* 5, 457–468.

Sheldrake, P. (1987) *Images of Holiness.* London: Darton, Longman and Todd.

Speck, P. (1988) *Being There: Pastoral Care in Time of Illness.* London: SPCK.

Stout, J. (1988) *Ethics after Babel.* Cambridge: James Clarke.

Taylor, J. (1972) *The Go-Between God.* London: SCM Press.

Wakefield, G. (ed) (1983) *A Dictionary of Christian Spirituality.* London: SCM Press.

Weber, M. (1963) *The Sociology of Religion.* Boston: Beacon Press.

Wink, W. (1984) *Naming the Powers.* Philadelphia: Fortress Press.

Witherington, B. (2000) *Jesus the Seer: The Progress of Prophecy.* Peabody (Mass.): Hendrickson Publishers.

Woodward, J. (1999) 'A Study of the Acute Health Care Chaplain in England.' Unpublished PhD dissertation of the Open University.

CHAPTER 3

Spiritual Institutions?

David Lyall

There are some conversations you can't help overhearing. It was a young man's voice I heard as I browsed through the books in the Mind and Spirit section of Waterstone's book shop in Tunbridge Wells. 'My girlfriend has decided to become a witch' (said the voice). 'It is quite easy you know. You just buy one of these books and all the rituals are there.' At that point I think I began to understand the meaning of postmodern, pick-and-mix, do-it-yourself spirituality.

I choose my words carefully. Some time ago at a meeting in our church offices, the word spirituality was introduced into a discussion at which another person added the words 'whatever that means', and for the rest of that meeting we spoke of the hyphenated 'spirituality-whatever-that-means'. 'Spirituality' is a word which no longer *has* a meaning. It is a word, a concept, onto which are projected many meanings, and the meaning which is given is largely a function of the experience and understanding of the person who bestows it.

The word 'spirituality' is one which has traditionally been applied to individuals, and within a generation this word in this arena has undergone massive development. It is a long way from the narrow concept of spirituality embodied, for example, in the figure of the ascetic spiritual director in Susan Howatch's novels about the Church of England to the much broader concepts contained in the books on Mind and Spirit which fill the shelves of even the general bookshops. If it is difficult to agree what spirituality is in relation to individuals, how much more in relation to institutions? In a recent article on 'Organisational Spirituality', Stephen Pattison (2000), in his usual perceptive way, appears to have said everything which can or needs to be said on the subject. However, as I have reflected on his paper, I have become aware of the same questions concerning the nature of organisational spirituality as I have about much of the contemporary discussion on individual spirituality. I will return to this paper in due course, but first let me say something about the use of the term by Peter Speck and then in the nursing literature.

Religious needs and spiritual needs

In his book *Being There*, Peter Speck (1988) did us all a service by pointing out the very real difference between the *spiritual* needs of patients and their *religious* needs. He points to the danger of chaplains rushing in to satisfy the religious needs of patients, whether these needs be expressed or perceived, when in fact to do so is to inhibit the expression and possible response to a deeper spiritual need. He tells the story of a chaplain being called to minister to a man whose daughter was on a life-support machine after crashing her moped. The man demanded that the chaplain pray for a miracle. The chaplain's refusal to respond as the man demanded led to a deeper relationship and exploration of the father's sense of guilt because he had bought the moped and given it to his daughter. Speck highlights the way in which the attempt to meet religious needs can prevent an exploration of deeper spiritual needs. He describes these needs as being related to:

- loss of meaning
- intense suffering
- a lack of a sense of the presence of God
- anger towards God or his perceived representatives
- a sense of guilt or shame
- a concern for the ethical issues involved in treatment
- unresolved feelings about death.

It is interesting, however, to note that in his differentiation between religious needs and spiritual needs, Speck produces a list of spiritual needs that are decidedly religious in their content. But then he is speaking as a chaplain in close touch with what patients actually say and, as we shall see, this is quite important.

The nursing literature presents a more varied understanding of the nature of spirituality. Thus Linda Ross defines the spiritual dimension as 'that element within the individual from which originates: meaning, purpose and fulfilment in life; a will to live; belief and faith in self, others and God and which is essential to the attainment of an optimum state of health, well-being or quality of life' (1997, p.11). A paper by Pamela Reed (1992) in *Research in Nursing and Health* explores 'An Emerging Paradigm in the Investigation of Spirituality in Nursing.' This article brings together material reflecting the burgeoning interest in spirituality in nursing. In her review of this literature she identifies a number of recurring themes, including those of interconnectedness and self-transcendence.

In contrast with Ross's paper, what emerges from Reed's analysis is that traditional understandings of the nature of God have no necessary place in spirituality as understood by nurses – or at least by those involved in nursing research. She concludes: 'Components of spirituality cross traditional science boundaries such that the *spiritual* cannot be distinguished necessarily from what has been labeled as the *social, psychological or physical* parts of a human being' (1992, p.354). Now, of course, behind this statement, there is much to celebrate in its understanding of what it means to be human. Nurses with a concern for spirituality as interconnectedness and transcendence will see patients as something other than broken-down machines. They will see patients in all their relatedness to others, to their inner selves and to whatever they believe lies beyond themselves. It is a celebration of the human spirit and here we have both its strength and its limitations. Its strength lies in its vision of the person as more than a machine; its limitation from a Christian perspective is that God becomes at best an optional extra, one particular mode of expression of the transcendent and a somewhat dated one at that.

In her more recent writing, Reed has developed a much more sophisticated (and arguably less reductionist) model of spirituality in relation to health care embracing both the heights and the depths of human experience and taking seriously the impact of postmodern ideas on our understanding of reality:

> Soul, from the Greek translation of soul as psyche, is linked most often to what today is referred to as the person's emotional experiences of awe, meaning, despair, suffering, joy and beauty. Soul is about depth, whereas spirit is about height. Spirit, from the Greek word 'pneuma', expresses connectedness to a creative power beyond the self, and equips one to commune with God and the spirits. (1998, p.43)

While one might wish to question the identification of soul with depth and spirit with height, nevertheless working with Reed's definitions and her understanding of the need to move beyond modern (as opposed to postmodern) understandings of the nature of reality there is room for a more traditional approach to spirituality.

> Health care praxis within this paradigm focuses on nurturing the patient's spirit and spiritual gifts. This may entail designing experiences and environments in which patients can commune with God, celebrate their relationship with God, and continue to grow spiritually. Allowing or creating time for patients to express spiritual needs or for receiving sacraments with clergy are also important practices within this paradigm. (Reed 1998, p.50)

In the contemporary debate about the meaning of spirituality, we see a reflection of the questions which have been at the heart of the Christological debates since Christians began to reflect upon their faith and the One who is at its centre. Who is this Jesus? Was he human or was he divine? These debates struggled with such issues, producing creeds and confessions which tried to safeguard truth as agreed by the Church as a whole. To understand the person of Jesus Christ in all his fullness, both his humanity and his divinity had to be affirmed and held in creative tension. The divinity and the humanity of Jesus Christ must neither be confused nor separated. Failure to do so resulted in what was perceived to be heresy.

In a sense there is a similar kind of process happening in the contemporary debate about spirituality. Speck has pointed to the fact that the religious and the spiritual are frequently collapsed into one another and there is a need to make a distinction between them. He does not, however, totally separate them and indeed his list of spiritual needs indicates that the religious may commonly be the expression of the spiritual. In a more recent publication he re-affirms this point:

> A wider understanding of the word spiritual, as relating to the search for existential meaning within any given life experience, allows us to consider spiritual needs and issues in the absence of any clear practice of religion or faith, but this does not mean that they are separated from each other. (Speck 1998, p.23)

The context of contemporary chaplaincy is precisely this tension between contemporary 'humanistic' understandings of spirituality and more traditional Christian approaches. I want to argue that within this context, the key issues in hospital chaplaincy relate to identity and integrity. There is undoubtedly much disillusionment with institutional religion and we must be sensitive to that. There is also growing evidence of the reality of religious experience as evidenced in the research of David Hay and Kate Hunt (2000). They have demonstrated in their 'Soul of Britain' survey that 76 per cent of the population admit to some kind of spiritual experience (a huge positive response compared with 25 years ago). They add:

> In these circumstances, the Church's major concern should not, in the first place, be about filling pews. The first thing is to observe how God is already communicating with these millions of people... If the soul of Britain is waking up, perhaps it is time for us to take notice. (p.846)

All this is true but it is not the whole truth. In the same issue of the journal in which Stephen Pattison's article appears there is another paper looking at 'Spiritual Perspectives among Terminally Ill Patients'. The significance of this study, carried out in 1998 in South Wales, is that almost universally there was an inability on the part of the patients to distinguish between spirituality and religion. The authors write:

> Perhaps there is a word of caution here for those who in their reasonable desire to widen the concept of spirituality in a pluralistic society, are in danger of severing it from its traditional forms of expression, divorcing religion (restrictive) from spirituality (open and free). (Ballard *et al.* 2000, p.30)

In the midst of such diversity, it is arguable, perhaps even obvious, that chaplains can only minister out of their own narrative. By this I mean that while chaplains must take note of the varied belief systems of the people to whom they minister, they can only minister out of their own centredness. By this I don't mean an exclusivist clinging to a rigid belief system that cannot be open to the other, but rather an identity located within a deeper kind of centredness that can affirm others on their particular pilgrimage. I suggest that it is only with this kind of personal spirituality, defined by its centre rather than its boundaries, that chaplains can function in the midst of the cultural and spiritual diversity which constitutes the modern hospital.

Can one speak of institutional spirituality?

What has all this to do with institutional spirituality? I want to argue that the critical issues in the debate about institutional spirituality are a reflection or recapitulation of those in the more familiar field of individual spirituality. But first a more basic question: is it at all appropriate to talk of institutional spirituality? Stephen Pattison clearly thinks it is. In his exploration of organisational spirituality, he draws upon the work of the New Testament scholar Walter Wink. He outlines a concept of organisational spirituality in terms of what he (and Wink) see as 'the inner aspect of material or tangible manifestations of power'(Wink 1984, p.104). In many ways, this spiritual or 'within' aspect of any power nexus, group or society acts as its character or personality by analogy with the individual person. In other words, institutions have a personality, a character, an inward disposition analogous to but separate from the individuals who form them. Are they right? What about congregations, surely the most spiritual of all organisations? Let me tell you about two congregations, both of which shall remain anonymous. I can think of one congregation which over the past 30 years or so has had a succession of four short but creative ministries from men (as it happens) in the first ministries. This congregation has had the knack of choosing young ministers, nurturing them in their early years, and sending them on their way to more demanding parishes. I know of another congregation which also had four ministries over the same period. Two of these ministers died in their early 50s and two moved on to become hospital chaplains. I think it must be recognised as a fact of life that some institutions – including churches – are life-enhancing and some are life-constricting. Sometimes a group of people, individually sane and well-balanced, in the group setting take on a group character which is quite destructive. And of course this can happen in any group or institution. Why this should be so is open to debate but detailed discussion falls beyond the scope of this paper.

And so I return to Stephen Pattison's paper. He begins by trying to visualise the hospital as an organisation in terms of an image that is significant for him. And for him that image is 'a picture of a wizened old man in a white coat sitting on his own in a room high in a tower and counting money with an avaricious expression on his worried face' (Pattison 2000, p.15). That image drives Pattison's understanding of the spirituality of the hospital as institution. Perhaps it is not a surprising image coming from the author of *The Faith of the Managers* (Pattison 1997). It leads to an understanding of the hospital in which the bottom line (his phrase) is financial. Now, money undoubtedly contributes to the ethos (spirituality?) of the modern NHS hospital. As he himself admits, other people will have different images. Indeed it is arguable that the very fact that people continue to work in the NHS and give themselves selflessly, means that they are driven by other more compelling images, images which express compassion and commitment. Or, indeed, that the situation is even more complex. In another important study Stephen Pattison has attempted to understand the values operating in the NHS by bringing people together, both staff and patients, to tell the stories of their interaction with the NHS. He elicited stories of courage and commitment beyond the call of duty. But there were other more disturbing stories, stories of power and abuse and depersonalisation, and of people demonstrating values in their work that were a direct contradiction of finer, personal values deeply held. Thus the organisation itself, and the contemporary pressures upon it and within it, generated a different kind of ethos from that which would have been espoused by the individuals within it (Pattison, Manning and Maltby 1999).

In truth the spirituality of an organisation such as a modern hospital is many-faceted. There are undoubtedly the attitudes and feelings generated through working in an institution that will never have all the resources to do what could be done. There are the motivations, Christian or otherwise, that find expression in a sense of vocation to work with the sick; there are all the understandings of spirituality that exist in contemporary society that find expression in the way people act when the chips are down. Among these understandings are the search for connectedness and the sense of that which transcends the self as identified in the nursing literature. Pattison identifies the need for ministry to the spirit of an organisation in a state of continuing uncertainty and change. He does not specify who might exercise this ministry but I assume that chaplains might have a contribution to make. What might be the parameters of such a ministry?

First there is the need to recognise the complex nature of contemporary spirituality. Spirituality can never be reduced to a 'nothing but...' phenomenon. There is always something more to be said. We will welcome the concern for connectedness as part of what it means to be authentically human. We will celebrate the discovery of the need for and the possibility of self-transcendence but in so doing we will ask whether *self*-transcendence exhausts all that needs to be said about transcendence. For at the heart of the Judaeo-Christian religion there is a belief in One who is Wholly Other, a transcendent Being who is much more than something beyond ourselves.

Spirituality as the search for right religion

Here I think we come to the heart of the matter. I want to take the risk of naming the spiritual task as the search for right religion. I speak of risk because I am well aware of the damage caused by the wrong kind of religion. Indeed one of the tasks of a chaplain may be to rid the hospital of the wrong kind of religion. On my first Sunday afternoon as a hospital chaplain, I arrived during visiting to find a service being broadcast throughout the hospital over the loudspeaker system. Up and down every corridor impinging upon the ears of the living and the dying, patients and visitors alike, came a badly sung version of 'Nearer My God to Thee'. The Matron asked nicely if this was really a good idea... Then came Christmas. I was told the chaplain always had Christmas dinner in the Radiotherapy Unit. So I presented myself at 12.30 to find the remaining 12 patients – all too ill to go home – propped up at a table with the chaplain and deaconess at the head of the table, everybody wearing fancy hats. The nursing staff called it 'The Last Supper'. It was certainly the last Christmas dinner we did that way.

At the end of the day, in the midst of the complexity of contemporary spirituality, individual and institutional, and all that passes for religion, good and bad, chaplains can only be who they are, representatives of a eucharistic, story-formed community. To be otherwise is simply to reflect the fragmentation of contemporary society and religion and be of little use to the hospital as institution. Yet this must be done with a certain discernment. I like to think of authentic spirituality as being secure at its centre but fuzzy at its boundaries.

Ten years after I began my chaplaincy – despite the bad image of religion that existed on my arrival and maybe because of our willingness to get rid of it – we opened a new Chaplaincy Centre in the hospital. It was funded partly by hospital endowments, partly by the WRVS, partly by churches and partly by voluntary effort on the part of many staff. It was a project that was owned by the hospital as an institution. While some senior staff wanted to build a chapel, the chaplaincy team – now ecumenical – held out for a chaplaincy centre and that is what we got, a multi-purpose building with a worship area, but also space for meetings and for meeting, for counselling and supervision.

At the centre of the worship area was a simple communion table and behind it a tapestry, which the artist called 'Clouds of Peace'. The extent to which it contained Christian symbolism lay in the eyes of the beholder.

At the heart of the life of the chapel we had Daily Prayers for ten minutes at lunch time, attended by the chaplaincy team when they were in, plus a regular group of staff and occasionally by patients and/or their families. Over the sandwich lunch which followed, the chaplains reviewed their morning's work together. Students on placement were part of that discussion and some claim that that is where they learned about ministry. Worship was held every Sunday and the communion services always seemed to be particularly significant. These were held once a month – rather frequent for Presbyterian Scotland but if I had stayed longer I think I might have bit the bullet and moved to every week. Why? Because the image of broken bread and shared wine spoke to people with broken bodies and whose blood was being shed during their stay in hospital. And because for many patients this was the first time they had taken communion in years – and for a few the first time ever. (Chaplains will recognise that pastoral practice drives a coach and horses through traditional sacramental theology – or, perhaps, forces us to reformulate our theology of the sacraments in the light of pastoral practice.)

While non-Christian groups would have been welcome to use the chaplaincy facilities, I am not aware of any that did so in my time. Why they did not do so could well provoke some discussion. Despite our efforts to be sensitive to the needs of others, it may still have been seen as a Christian space. The hospital as an institution did however make every effort to be sensitive to the religious needs of other faith groups such as the ritualistic washing of bodies after a death had taken place.

I am arguing therefore that on the one hand, chaplains must recognise the complexity of the spirituality that pervades an institution such as the modern hospital. And I am arguing, on the other hand, that chaplains can only minister to this complexity out of the integrity of their own narrative. Is there not a contradiction here? I think not. It is when ministry comes out of the particularity of an individual narrative that it has most universal appeal. Rabbi Lionel Blue, with his inimitable brand of story-telling, is the only religious person who can speak to me – and I suspect many others – before eight o'clock in the morning. Similarly, Thomas Merton is now recognised as someone who has had a profound influence upon our contemporary understanding of spirituality. While he spent most of his adult life in the monastery, he was no recluse shut off from the realities of the world. From his hermitage he sought for what was most authentically human. He was involved in the campaign for civil rights; he sought dialogue with Christians who were not Catholics and with monks who were not Christian. Yet in all this interaction with the principalities and powers, Merton never ceased to be who he was – a Christian, a Catholic, a monk and a priest. Rooted with integrity in his own identity, he could with equal integrity work from his own centredness to embrace the rich diversity of humankind.

Amidst the complexity of the spirituality which pervades the modern hospital, a pastoral ministry rooted in the narratives of communities of faith, nurtured by the rituals and symbols of these communities, and open to the spiritual needs of people and places, is well worth aiming for.

References

Ballard, P., Finlay, I., Jones, N., Searle, C. and Roberts, S. (2000) 'Spiritual Perspectives Among Terminally Ill Patients.' *Modern Believing 41*, 2, 30–38.

Hay, D. and Hunt, K. (2000) 'Is Britain's Soul Waking Up?' *The Tablet* 24 June, p.846.

Pattison, S. (1997) *The Faith of the Managers.* London: Cassell.

Pattison, S., Manning, S. and Malby, B. (1999) 'I want to tell you a story.' *Health Service Journal* 28 February, p.22–24.

Pattison, S. (2000) 'Organizational spirituality: an exploration.' *Modern Believing 41*, 2, 12–20.

Reed, P. G. (1992) 'An emerging paradigm for the investigation of spirituality in nursing.' *Research in Nursing and Health 15*, 349–357.

Reed, P.G. (1998) 'The re-enchantment of health care.' In M. Cobb and V. Robshaw (eds) *The Spiritual Challenge of Health Care.* Edinburgh: Churchill Livingstone.

Ross, L. A. (1997) *Nurses' Perception of Health Care.* Aldershot: Avebury.

Speck, P. (1988) *Being There: Pastoral Care in Times of Illness.* London: SPCK.

Speck, P. (1998) 'The meaning of spirituality in illness.' In M. Cobb and V. Robshaw (eds) *The Spiritual Challenge of Health Care.* Edinburgh: Churchill Livingstone.

Wink, W. (1984) *Naming the Powers.* Minneapolis: Fortress.

CHAPTER 4

Discerning the Spirits

Theological Audit in Health Care Organisations

Margaret Whipp

Audit and change

The process of audit is defined by the Oxford English Dictionary as 'a searching examination (especially the day of judgement)'. Perhaps it is not surprising, then, that the introduction of audit into health care organisations has been seen as quite a challenge. Whether it is the relentless scrutiny of outpatient waiting times, or the rigorous visitation of an accreditation inspectorate, the potential of audit as a force for change is recognised in every sphere of health care activity. Audit holds up a mirror to professionals in their practice, to processes in their performance, within which the reality of care in the service is brought sharply into focus. In this chapter, I will develop the notion of 'theological audit' (Challen 1996) to suggest ways in which the spiritual realities that shape a health care organisation might be examined and brought to account as forces for change.

Discernment, and a searching examination of conscience, are disciplines well known within the tradition of Christian spiritual care. In the spiritual direction of individuals, and in the guidance of Christian communities, it is not unusual to apply quite structured and methodical techniques to bring into conscious reflection those underlying spiritual and theological principles which move and motivate the practical outworkings of faith. By unearthing and articulating these principles, it becomes possible to imagine new paths of faithfulness.

Commitment to change is an essential prerequisite. Some years ago, a triad of Christian professionals committed to work together over a six-month period to examine the forces that were distorting the quality of care in each of three hospital departments. Taking Walter Wink's approach to 'unmasking the powers', they tried to penetrate beneath the surface of dysfunctional professional groups to the deeper spiritual principles that affected their work (cf. Wink 1983 and 1986). One by one, they named the unspoken fears that blocked effective patient care: fear of change, fear of inadequacy, fear of burn out, fear of bullying. As individuals, and together in mutual support, they struggled to shape new strategies that could counter a climate of fear, and encourage a fresh spirit of compassion. Through the discipline of theological audit, they grew in confidence as reflective practitioners, and as resourceful leaders of patient-centred care.

Imagination and transformation

Christians have a powerful impetus for transformation. *Metanoia* is the New Testament word for conversion. It denotes a change of mind, a re-shaping of perspectives in the light of the searching judgement of God and the glorious hope of his Kingdom. Thus, St Paul urges Christians to be transformed by the renewal of their minds. By cultivating a theologically informed imagination, they are to be empowered as agents of change and eschatological transformation amid the conflicts of everyday life. 'Then,' explains St Paul, 'you will be able to discern the will of God, and to know what is good, acceptable and perfect' (Romans 12:2).

Dynamic models of theology revel in the positive processes of change and development. Rather than seeking spiritual reassurance in unchanging formulations of past experience, they take transformation seriously, pursuing every possibility of hope and renewal through a radical imagination of how things might become. The God of the process theologians is a re-engineering God.

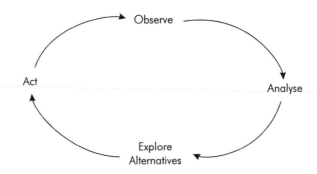

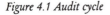
Figure 4.1 Audit cycle

This active commitment to 'do theology' (Green 1990) in practical contexts is not far removed from the vision of audit as a tool for continuous improvement that has been taken up so avidly by the proponents of quality management. Though one is spiritually inspired and the other entirely secular, both are rigorous disciplines, inspired by radical hope.

As a model of change, the audit cycle can be conceived as a series of discrete steps, as shown in Figure 4.1.

1. *Observation* begins the process of change. Typically, what might be observed is a failure to care. This may be measured quantitatively against some statistical gauge of adequacy. Or, more subtly, qualitative observations seek to articulate the shape of what is missing in the overall experience of patient care. Where is healing being thwarted? How is justice being denied?

2. *Analysis* is the crucial step for critical discernment. What values are operating, and how can they be named? Which criteria apply, and for what purpose? Who holds power in the situation, and who is excluded from power? Where are the blocks to genuine care, and what is keeping those blocks in place?

3. *Explore alternatives.* An element of playfulness is good at this point. To release the imagination, it is important to feel free to be creative in re-designing different approaches to care. Alternatives need to be bold, but also realistic. What is most important here? What might make all the difference? What can be honestly achieved and sustained? And, vitally, who will do it?

4. *Act.* The weakness of many audit initiatives is revealed in a final failure of nerve. The transformation that is imagined must be put into practice, even if that practice is only a provisional plan. Indeed, if the audit cycle is to continue, it is important that outcomes are not cast in stone too quickly before further scrutiny has evaluated their effectiveness. Better an honest mistake than the paralysing fear of further failure. Positive action, however preliminary, is the essential outcome for an effective audit cycle.

The complete audit cycle, as it has been developed for quality management, is a highly effective tool for improving operational aspects of patient care. That much is to be expected from a model drawn from manufacturing industry. The challenge for spiritual care practitioners is to forge equally effective tools for a theological interrogation of the practice of health care.

Among the deeper issues for an organisation to examine are the spiritual issues of motivation and value and quality of care. They are the forces, above and beyond the more measurable criteria of successful care which might be investigated with a very clear focus through carefully designed theological audit.

Theological audit is offered as a tool for critical development of the spiritual foundations on which a caring organisation is founded. Every organisation holds spiritual values and criteria deeply embedded within its culture. Each act of patient care is powerfully influenced by the norms embodied within the organisation and enacted, often unconsciously, by those who work within it.

I suggest, therefore, an approach to theological audit in health care organisations that has four critical aims: *to make values explicit, to make criteria clear, to make choices accountable* and *to make change imaginable.*

Cultivating reflection

Reflective practice is now a recognised aspect of professional accountability in a range of clinical and managerial contexts (Schon 1983). Based on action-reflection models of adult learning, individuals and teams are encouraged to expand their skills and knowledge through the practice of personal or group reflection on experiences of professional life. In this section, I will outline a few practical methods for using the approach of reflective practice as a basis for theological audit.

1. Personal journalling

As an accessible introduction to theological audit, journal exercises are an invigorating tool for development. Based on classic spiritual exercises such as the Ignatian examination of consciousness, journal exercises can develop a keener understanding of values and a warmer appreciation of the motivation to care.

One group of hospital staff chose to reflect on Matthew Fox's 'Spirituality of Work Questionnaire' (Fox 1994). Crucial questions touched on creativity and pain, challenge and motivation for those involved in both direct and indirect patient care.

Exploring such questions is only a first step into theological audit. Ongoing work with an individual's journal can lead to anything from 'the gentle probing of discipleship at work to the severe and willing reappraisal

Do I experience joy in my work?

- *When, and under what circumstances?*
- *How often?*
- *How can the joy be increased?*
- *How does this joy relate to the pain and difficulties at work?*

When did I first feel drawn to the kind of work I am doing?

- *What did it feel like?*
- *Has this feeling increased or decreased over the years?*
- *Have I lost touch with this feeling over the years?*
- *How can this feeling be regenerated?*

How am I emptied at work?

- *How does nothingness happen at my work?*
- *What is my response to nothingness at work?*

What am I doing to reinvent the profession in which I work?

- *How am I bringing justice, compassion, and celebration to the world by way of my work?*
- *How am I returning my profession to its origins as a sacred or sacramental work?*

(Fox 1994, Appendix 1)

Figure 4.2 Some questions for a spirituality of work

of professional responsibilities' (Challen 1996, p.144). Alternatively, a group of co-professionals, whether or not united by a common faith, may commit together to the outworking of such a spiritual analysis in a radical review of their shared patterns of care.

2. Value clarification

Reflective skills are an important quality to develop in health care professionals whose training has focused more on the physical and economic sciences than on the human and social sciences. With careful facilitation, it is encouraging to see how the incisive analytical skills of clinicians and managers can be directed towards a critical reflection on roles and responsibilities within an ethical and spiritual framework.

A workshop for budget holders in a medium-sized Trust explored the roles that had to be enacted in the allocation of scarce resources. In order to heighten their awareness of the spiritual and ethical dimensions, each role was labelled with a biblical description.

The *steward* is someone who is responsible and accountable for the development and administration of resources that are not his or her own. She needs to be honest about the limits of her capacities, and unselfish in the way she manages them. The steward may be accountable in several directions at once. In a hospital, there will be accountability towards commissioning authorities to set alongside the accountability to immediate patient care. When these accountabilities come into conflict, the steward bears the strain.

The *scapegoat* is someone who bears a load for everyone else, especially when things go wrong. Inevitably, in human organisations and processes, failures and frustrations will play a part. The scapegoat's responsibility is to carry the can for this, not evading the painful realities of human limitations, but taking the trouble and bearing the pain. When ideals confront actualities, the scapegoat has a tough time, but if he can bear the burden graciously, he becomes an agent of real salvation for others.

The *shepherd* is someone who upholds the personal significance of our corporate endeavours. He is not charged with impersonal balance sheets, but rather with the care of the flock (perhaps of patients, staff or students), attentive to each individual need. It is the shepherd's responsibility to look out for them, in fair weather or foul, to lead them to good pastures, and to rescue them from danger. He takes care of their weaknesses, carrying the lambs in his arms. He also encourages their strengths, encouraging the able sheep to get on and walk. In all this, the shepherd embraces this personal responsibility, not for the reward of a hireling's wage, but because he loves the sheep as his own.

The *seer* is someone charged with taking the long view of the situation. Her responsibility is not to collude with short-term, pragmatic decisions, but to urge the priority of unseen consequences for the future common good. The seer cannot be too loyal to the here and now. She must be big and brave enough to overturn orthodoxy and assert counter-cultural values. As dreamers of dreams, seers are often accused of fecklessness and naivety.

Sitting loose to the political slogans of the moment, they are not infrequently marginalised or misunderstood.

Alongside a confidential mentor, each budget manager was invited to claim the role most appropriate to their current responsibility, and to explore the ethical challenges and motivations that touched upon their daily experience. The result was an intense identification with the ideological conflicts and spiritual temptations suggested by the biblical role models. Shabby and pragmatic compromises were exposed in the light of the value clarity that arose from the theological context. In each participant, a sense of moral consciousness was re-awakened, and the support and stimulation of the group facilitated serious commitments to specific change. Many months later, the effects of the audit were still apparent when budget holders commiserated with the 'scapegoat' in their midst, or encouraged the 'seer' to think the unthinkable whatever the immediate reaction. Role identification, together with value clarification, led to new courage and confidence in ethical decision making.

3. Narrative exploration

A third practical example of an approach to theological audit adopts a narrative approach. I am indebted to the work of Stephen Pattison for elucidating the value of storytelling as a resource for discernment in an action-reflection methodology.

> Stories offer us a way in to seeing living values or values in action. A story calls upon us to identify with it, and this process changes us by prompting us to re-interpret our views, to re-think the impact of our actions. Whilst our response to a story tells us something about ourselves, sharing our responses moves us beyond where we are. (Maltby and Pattison 1999, p.41)

The point of a story-telling workshop is to explore values in practice. There is frequently a discrepancy, especially in an ideologically rich organisation such as the NHS, between values that are espoused and values that are enacted. The risk of talking about values in an abstract way is that only noble and acceptable values may be owned. Health care staff are then left struggling with an unsatisfactory feeling that worthy values cannot hold up in practice. They are unable to 'walk the talk'. The point of a story-telling session is to reckon with actual values in practice.

In a King's Fund project for the NHS's 50th year, NHS staff, managers and service users were invited to participate in story-telling workshops. Each participant was asked to contribute their own 'defining moment' story from the past few years. These might include experiences with patients, relationships with colleagues, situations where they had to make a hard decision, moments of realisation that the NHS does not work in quite the way they had thought it did, and their own experience as a user (Maltby and Pattison 1999).

The result was a telling piece of analysis, in which the lived and enacted values could be interrogated and set alongside the alleged values of care which the NHS, in theory, subscribes to – values such as equality of access, putting patients first, being caring, and valuing individuals and their differences. Stories were told of gross discrepancies in care – between London and the provinces, between children and adults, between the acute sick and those with long-term disabilities. Painful stories were told to illustrate offensive attitudes – the arrogance of doctors, the lack of patient-centredness and unwillingness to listen, whilst other heartening stories related a heroic commitment to the care of patients, even when the patients were difficult and disruptive. Critical stories revealed the contrast between caring facilities for patients versus oppressive and uncaring attitudes to the staff who provide those facilities.

As a timely audit, the King's Fund project provided a snapshot journalist's view of the spiritual state of the NHS in its 50th year. Caring values that were deeply embedded in the espoused culture of the NHS were inspected in practice, and found wanting:

Let's all introduce ourselves and tell each other tales,
About who we know's been crucified,
And what they used for nails.
About wheeler-dealer politics, what your job title is today,
And who remembers the little things,
And on whose side it's best to play.
'Always tell the truth,' she said.
A fanciful idea she'd had taught her.
I don't think I'll be trying it,
'Til I've learnt to walk on water.

(Maltby and Pattison 1999, i)

It would be unworkable in the context of a one-day workshop for delegates from different health care settings to drive the audit cycle towards exploration of alternatives and positive action. In local groups, however, a story-telling workshop can become a springboard for significant change. One mixed group of health care and other professionals used story-telling as a basis for strengthening their discipleship in working life. After a story-telling session on power, in which forms of power and its abuse were critically analysed, they each contributed a story on transformation, in which opportunities to overturn abuses of power were eagerly related. The support of the audit group had facilitated a process of change and a new spirit of justice.

4. Implementing the audit cycle

The above examples have been chosen to illustrate some approaches to reflection that have been simply and successfully applied within health care settings. These methods and many others may be accessible ways to introduce theological audit as an aspect of spiritual care for individuals and entire organisations. In most cases, it will be feasible only to facilitate one part of the complete audit cycle (see figure 4.1, p.58).

Initially, any opportunity for observation and comment alone may be sufficient to trigger a change of outlook. Beyond that, thoughtful analysis and clarification of ethical and spiritual and theological dimensions of care can be astonishingly fruitful. Educational programmes and professional development projects are increasingly alive to more reflective approaches to learning, in which the role of a spiritual care professional as facilitator can be immensely helpful. For the full audit cycle to take effect, however, there must be some exploration and implementation of action for change. This is inevitably the most challenging point of the audit cycle, where the people observing and analysing and making recommendations may not be the same people, or may not have the same power, or may hold different value commitments from the people who put recommendations into action. The reality of an ethically pluralistic context found in health care organisations means that an agreed basis for change cannot be assumed. An audit described as *theological* audit, offered as a set of tools in support of organisational development, may be perceived in some secular contexts as inappropriately threatening or imperialistic. The integrity of the spiritual care professional, who uses his or her skills of discernment to serve the wider good of an ethically diverse community, lies in contributing a theologically inspired critique to a many-sided debate about the meaning and practice of care.

In the final section of this chapter, by way of a germane example, I take the concept of *care* itself as a subject for an extended reflection. Within the secular setting of most health care organisations, how might a theologically informed spiritual care professional contribute to a deeper understanding and truer praxis of authentic care?

The criterion of care

Presuppositions about the meaning of *care* lie at the heart of any significant debate within health care organisations. Whatever form of scrutiny is brought into play, whether scientific or economic or even theological, there is a criterion of care at the base of all our judgements by which the value of any type of health care activity is instinctively measured. Yet *care* itself remains very difficult to define precisely. An act of care might range from something as practical as providing prompt access to a properly fitted wheelchair to something as personal and intangible as the pastoral care offered to grief-stricken families in a hospice. Humanly speaking, there is a fundamentally common sense by which we recognise when care has been given, and – more sharply – when it has not.

In a delightful monograph entitled *On Caring*, Milton Mayeroff subjected the concept of care to a philosophical analysis. In conclusion he found that 'the meaning of caring is not to be confused with wishing well, liking, comforting and maintaining or simply having an interest in what happens to another. Caring, as helping another grow…is a process, a way of relating to someone that involves development' (1971, p.41).

Mayeroff identified eight essential components of caring:

- **Knowledge.** To care I must understand the other's need. This involves explicit and implicit knowledge.

- **Alternating rhythms**, alternating between interacting with others and reflecting on the consequences of the interaction.

- **Patience**. Not simply waiting for things to happen, but enabling others to grow in their own time and style.

- **Honesty**. Active openness and confrontation with oneself and others.

- **Trust**, appreciating the independent existence of others and allowing them to grow in their own way.

- **Humility**. Being willing to learn from others and be aware of one's own limitations.

- **Hope**. The possibility of something worthy of commitment.

- **Courage**. Makes risk taking possible. Founded in trust of one's own and the other's ability to grow.

(pp.8ff.)

Mayeroff suggests that caring is a value which orders all other values around it. It gives meaning to life, and enables each human person to find a place of belonging in the world.

Theological sources of care

The received Western tradition of care is rooted very deeply in Judeo-Christian theological concepts. The text from Matthew's Gospel – 'when I was hungry, you gave me food; when thirsty, you gave me a drink; when I was a stranger, you took me into your home; when naked, you clothed me; when I was ill, you came to my help; when in prison, you visited me' – is quoted over the portals of countless infirmaries and institutions throughout the Western world (Matthew 25:35-36). The list of caring actions depicted by Jesus was drawn, in turn, from Isaiah (Isaiah 58:6-7), and to that list the church added a final act, the burial of the dead, to form the seven Corporal Works of Mercy which have been foundational for the tradition of care for 20 centuries.

The vocation to care is inspired within the Christian tradition by an inexhaustibly caring image of God. Indeed there is a reckless profligacy in Christian narratives of care that exalt the unbounded generosity of One who embraces the prodigal, and touches the leper. Risk-taking, rule-breaking and boundary-stretching behaviour are characteristic of the 'good news' of genuinely Christian altruistic caring, expressed within a gift relationship in which the motive for care is not related to any expectation of reward.

There must be limits to care, however, when human beings who are themselves needy and broken become in turn, 'wounded healers' (Nouwen 1994). Their care is always partial and penultimate, never complete and without limitations of time or knowledge or skill. Thus, Alastair Campbell writes of 'moderated love' as the model for a professional stance of caring which gives freely of one's self *as far as that self is able* (1984).

Authentic care must be sustained on a secure base of loving relationships. Christian theology based on an inter-animating and Trinitarian experience of God understands that caring always springs from a prior source of love. Sustained, motivated, inspired by a God who *is* love, the Christian community seeks to embody that love and care within its corporate structures and institutions.

Practical problems of care

How successful can any institution be in putting a professed value of care into action? Theological critique can be usefully applied alongside other critical readings of everyday practice in evaluating the denials of care that daily undermine the identity and mission of organisations committed to health care.

The burden of caring, in practice, is frequently shrugged off. Energies are deflected elsewhere, into convenient distractions in the shape of reorganisations and relocations. Costs are shunted elsewhere, as budgets are relentlessly squeezed and secretly shuffled. Decisions are deferred elsewhere, as overburdened individuals blame the system or the management or the department next door. Those who do bear the burden are often left feeling isolated and unsupported in a climate where unremitting change undermines the only networks of support which might sustain their loving endeavours. Others merely pretend to care, hiding vested interests behind the professional persona that distances them from others, damaging and distorting the empathic relationships that are intrinsic to loving, personal care (cf Fox 1995).

A theological reflection on these everyday challenges to care reveals a spiritual deficiency at source. Care cannot be dispensed that has not first been resourced. 'We love because he (God) first loved us' (1 John 4:19). A theological audit of the shortfall in caring in contemporary health care organisations must focus on the spiritual springs from which the wells of caring might be renewed. What can be offered to an organisation and its staff to re-energise their vision, to refresh their jaded resources, to replenish their reserves of patience and hope and tender loving care? Spiritual care professionals, discerning the spirits of weariness and confusion in a service groaning under the burden of insatiable demands for care, might offer the simple gifts of joy and appreciation as appropriate tokens of a hoped-for transformation.

Care for the caring organisation

Theological audit is presented in this chapter as one form of active discernment which might be developed by spiritual care professionals entrusted with making a spiritual contribution to the common good of a secular health care institution.

At its simplest, it is an approach to the pastoral cycle based on action and reflection which can be helpful to use as a mental map when making sense of the challenges to care that are faced day by day. In its more developed form, the stages of the theological audit cycle can be used to give clarity to more serious and sustained efforts to probe the collective conscience of an organisation and facilitate some growth towards integrity and spiritual renewal.

Nothing may be assumed when 'theology' is applied within a 'secular' context. There is no explicit covenant of care founded on shared theological understandings of sacred covenant. Yet by unearthing the deeper spiritual bedrocks on which any caring foundation must be built, the theological auditor can facilitate new security and resilience within the complex fabric of human attitudes and relationships that bear the strain of the daily attempt to care.

References

Biblical quotations are taken from the *Revised English Bible* (1990). Cambridge University Press.

Campbell, A. (1984) *Moderated Love: A Theology of Professional Care.* London: SPCK.

Challen, P. (1996) 'Theological Audit - Interpreted and Applied Theology.' In J. W. Rogerson (ed) *Industrial Mission in a Changing World.* Sheffield: Academic Press.

Fox, M. (1994) *The Reinvention of Work: A New Vision of Livelihood for Our Time.* New York: Harper Collins.

Fox, N. (1995) 'Postmodern perspectives on care: the vigil and the gift.' *Critical Social Policy 15,* 107-125.

Green, L. (1990) *Let's Do Theology - A Pastoral Cycle Resource Book.* London: Mowbray.

Maltby, B. and Pattison, S. (1999) *Living Values in the NHS: Stories from the NHS's Fiftieth Year.* London: King's Fund Publishing.

Mayeroff, M. (1971) *On Caring.* New York: Perennial Library; Harper Collins.

Nouwen, H. (1994) *The Wounded Healer.* London: Darton, Longman and Todd.

Schon, D. A. (1983) *The Reflective Practitioner: How Professionals Think in Action.* London: Temple Smith.

Wink, W. (1983) *Naming the Powers: The Language of Power in the New Testament.* Philadelphia: Fortress Press.

Wink, W. (1986) *Unmasking the Powers: The Invisible Forces that Determine Human Existence.* Philadelphia: Fortress Press.

PART TWO

Professional Contexts

CHAPTER 5

Walking on Water?

The Moral Foundations of Chaplaincy

Mark Cobb

> Vicki Gilbert was diagnosed with a malignant bone tumour in 1992, and as a result underwent 3 operations to remove most of her shinbone, her knee and to fit a titanium implant. She then underwent chemotherapy, but less than a year later she was informed that the diagnosis was wrong and that she had in fact had a harmless cyst. By this stage, her leg implant caused constant stress fractures and pain, and she had to have her leg amputated above the knee in September 1996. The unnecessary chemotherapy caused permanent damage to her kidneys for which she still takes medication, and which has left her with reduced sensation in her hands and feet, as well as damage to her hearing. Vicki Gilbert won a £1.2m settlement at the end of October of this year following a seven-year legal battle. (Dyer 2000, p.5)

It is self-evident that many medical interventions can be more harmful than helpful: drugs can be poisonous and surgery in any other context would be considered a form of grievous bodily harm. But when used for the benefit of the patient, particularly in sustaining and protecting life, such interventions, whatever harm they may unintentionally cause, are considered morally and legally defensible. In the case of Vicki Gilbert, early clinical errors that went unchecked precipitated a chain of incorrectly informed decisions that had disastrous consequences and which contravened the injunction enshrined in the Hippocratic Oath to abstain from intentionally harming, injuring or abusing the patient.

Complaints, malpractice litigation and public inquiries are a familiar feature of contemporary health care, encouraged by an empowered health consumer with high expectations. News stories about the latest miraculous cure or medical advance sit alongside stories of patient neglect and murderous doctors. But behind the big headlines are some very serious issues for the health service, many of which have an ethical nature. Consequently what have been considered acceptable conventional practices now appear to be inadequate or plainly immoral – the Bristol Inquiry and the retention of organs following post-mortems provides one such far-reaching example.

Health care chaplains, unlike many of their colleagues, may escape such scrutiny because of their low visibility, insignificant numbers and a perception that their role is relatively benign. But is there any reason to accept that the prevalence of unethical practice is any lower among chaplains than their colleagues in other health care disciplines? Chaplains are not involved in invasive procedures, nor are they responsible for clinical decisions that may have fatal outcomes, but they do work among vulnerable patients and with aspects of people's lives that can be intimate and fragile. Incompetence, abuse of trust or the violation of boundaries in these circumstances can have devastating consequences and inflict life-long damage.

A recent case involving a registered nurse should set alarm bells ringing with many chaplains. Anne Steele is a Christian who has been a self-professed evangelist for more than 30 years. She trained as a registered nurse 11 years ago. The case involves a patient who was suffering from fainting spells and was being cared for by Mrs Steele. She believed that evil spirits were making the patient ill and so she attempted to perform an exorcism. The patient got up to leave but fell to the floor. Instead of helping her up, Mrs Steele stood over her, allegedly saying, 'I rebuke you evil spirits, get thee from her body so she will be well.' Mrs Steele later commented, 'I was regarded as having stepped over the line by praying with the patient, but research has shown that it is part of a nurse's role to pray with the patient if they request it and agree to it.'

The UK Central Council for Nursing found Anne Steele guilty of serious professional misconduct. The Council's director said, 'Registered nurses are entitled to have strongly held religious and spiritual views, but they must not inflict their beliefs and practices on their patients, and they must never substitute those practices for professional nursing care' (Rumbelow 2000).

There is no equivalent Central Council for Chaplains, nor any specific statutory regulations. The College of Health Care Chaplains' Code of Professional Conduct cannot fill one side of A4 and runs to a derisory 12 clauses. For a discipline that might be presumed to champion moral probity and the good of the patient, there is little to demonstrate that its own moral foundations are adequate or its practices ethical. Is there a secure moral ground for health care chaplains or are they attempting to walk on water?

Why morality should matter to chaplains

The paucity of contemporary literature concerning ethical practice in health care chaplaincy could suggest that it is either irrelevant or that it can be somehow assumed. Both these propositions are troubling because it is just such complacent conditions that hold the potential for damaging practice. Health care is dependent upon fundamental moral obligations that allow patients to put their trust in others. Chaplains cannot operate outside of this moral commitment: they have no dispensation from the ethical demands we impose upon other health care disciplines, and they have no mandate to act in ways that avoid public scrutiny. If chaplaincy is to claim an implicit morality then this will need to be demonstrated and justified, for chaplains cannot expect others to know what this is. In either case, health care is a dynamic context, the knowledge and evidence base is progressing and new moral dilemmas are regularly presenting themselves. All this points towards the need for chaplains to carefully examine the moral justification for their actions, to consider the boundaries within which they work, and to articulate their understanding alongside other disciplines so that it may be understood, developed and where necessary, corrected.

If we take patient care to be a core task of chaplaincy, then a central moral focus will be the nature and basis of personal encounters. Morality is fundamental to our understanding of persons, and guides the way we behave towards one another. Even if not explicit, a chaplain operates within a moral framework that generates particular obligations and commitments, and because chaplains refer to patients as persons, as opposed to say disordered biochemistry, then the way the person is viewed will be pivotal to the moral orientation of the relationship. Again, should we not expect chaplains of all disciplines to be concerned with matters of human dignity and to 'believe', as one moral theologian states, 'that we ought to refrain from certain kinds of harms to others, because these sorts of harms are inconsistent with an acknowledgement of the value and worth of the human person' (Porter 1995, p.55)?

Chaplains may not be in a position to kill a patient through the administration of the wrong medication, but they could, for example, through misunderstanding a situation, disclose confidential information or, through being unaware of transference, reinforce a neurotic dependence. These in themselves may not constitute malpractice, but they could have significant consequences for someone and impede their well-being. Good intentions are inadequate when dealing with other people's lives, as is the naive optimism that what chaplains do is probably, at worst, benign. Health care chaplains ought to carry out their duties in ways that are morally deliberate and critically self-reflective in order to move beyond prejudices, self-interests and the unexamined claims and expectations of others.

Morality should matter to chaplains because they should be concerned to demonstrate their integrity in acting for the good of those they care for, particularly given the freedom that most chaplains enjoy. It should also matter because health care chaplains enter into relationships of care with people because of their role and duties, and these oblige them to act with greater moral sensitivity than, say, an ordinary member of the public. Being a health care chaplain is also different from being a minister of religion in the community, because although it can be argued that both have a general obligation to help those in need, and both may be expected to demonstrate concern and compassion, it is the chaplain who has made a commitment to act primarily on behalf of those who are ill and injured. It is the chaplain therefore who is bound by more specific responsibilities within the health care context and these have a different ethical character than those of the community minister.

The responsible and professional chaplain

Responsibility is central to our moral thinking. It is a concept that is fundamental to our relationships, and it enables us to put our trust in those we do not know. To be responsible means in general to be reliable and to be accountable for decisions, actions and omissions. It is a term commonly used to signify moral probity in that a responsible person can be entrusted with important matters because they have the ability and authority to deliberate and perform the right course of action. Responsibility can also be associated with a role in that certain offices are accorded particular duties and carry particular obligations.

Chaplains generally have a duty to provide spiritual care and with this duty they acquire certain authority and responsibility. Most chaplains have a dual responsibility, one to their employing Trust and one to their licensing or commissioning faith community. These responsibilities are detailed by the Trust in a contract and job description and by the faith community through a licence or similar authorisation. Ordained chaplains are also considered to hold a distinctive office as ministers of religion, and are usually therefore subject to more rigorous accountability. In the Church of England, for example, those in Holy Orders are held responsible for such things as the breach of the laws ecclesiastical; for neglect or inefficiency in the performance of the duties of their office; and for conduct inappropriate or unbecoming to their office (General Synod 2000). This is the closest chaplains get to professional regulation, although it is not consistent across faith communities. And if such accountability seems burdensome, it needs repeating that health care chaplains are uniquely authorised to work among highly vulnerable people and with aspects of their lives that are intimate and sacred. The responsibilities of this office require a distinctive moral commitment primarily to ensure that harm, which could easily be inflicted, is avoided and that the trust required to serve what we may term 'the spiritual good' of the patient is warranted and sustained.

The relationship of the chaplain to the patient takes on a distinctive ethical character because of the specific duties involved – duties that are not attributed to, but are sometimes claimed by, other health care disciplines, for example by the nurse Anne Steele. Indeed, if it was a chaplain instead of a nurse who had been before a disciplinary hearing over the same case I suspect that whilst a different argument would have been used the outcome would have been the same. In looking at chaplaincy from the moral perspective of responsibility we see that there are specific duties, distinctive functions and a commitment to act on behalf of the good of others. These bring us close to what may be considered the ethical grounds for professional practice. This is a concept that some clergy resist on the basis that they were ordained to *be* a priest or pastor and not to *do* a job. But presumably pastors and priests have a vocation to exercise some form of practical ministry and that functions and duties are never far away from ministry.

Despite confusion between professionalisation and professional identity, objections persist that the notion of a professional is incompatible with a ministry that deals with the spiritual. But it is surely unethical that spiritual care should be abandoned to unskilled, naive and unaccountable practice. Unprofessional practice is certainly not what the NHS is expecting in an age of clinical governance. Chaplains are distinctive because of their training, commitments, responsibilities and functions, and while these may translate for some into social status and power, these do not necessarily follow. However, there are more robust challenges against professions other than those of privilege: first and most notably is the obvious fact that professionals do cause harm and sometimes quite deliberately; second, the claims of difference by professionals may substantially be derived from ideologies that justify monopolies and self-interest rather than the benefit of those they serve; and third, it is unclear how we define a professional and what membership of a profession means.

The legitimate ground of professional ethics, according to the philosopher Daryl Koehn, is a largely unconditional public commitment by those who seek to promote the particular good of others. For example, lawyers and clergy pledge to fulfil the duties of their office in order to benefit those in need. The public declaration provides an assurance to those who may need them that their interests will be the primary focus of the relationship and it obliges professionals to be responsible for them. And because professional roles are in the public domain there is a reasonable expectation of what these entail and therefore a general sense of account-ability to more than the individual. Professionals, however, retain the discretion to act in the best interest of those they serve but to do so within certain limits, for trust implies limits. Koehn argues that professions merit trust: first, 'because they do not authorize the professional to subvert client values'; and second, because, 'they do not purport to do what they cannot do'(1994, p.177). On these two grounds alone the nurse, Anne Steele, was culpable of professional misconduct.

I am suggesting that, from a moral point of view, chaplains occupy a role that is consistent with the description of the professional, and can therefore find legitimate moral grounds for a professional practice, authority and responsibility. A professional ethic should also be important to chaplains because it is one that operates through personal encounters, respects individuality, promotes an unconditional approach and recognises the voluntary nature of the relationship. Chaplaincy without such an ethic is on less secure ground, is likely to justify less trust, and will depend more upon the compelling personalities of particular chaplains than on the dependable moral commitment of an office holder.

Pellegrino and Thomasma contend that there are four fundamental features of a healing and helping profession: the nature of the human needs it addresses; the vulnerable state of those it serves; the expectations of trust it generates; and the social contract it implies (1997, p.91). These charac-teristics present substantive reasons for the moral obligations demanded of professionals who care for the ill and injured. They also differentiate roles undertaken for contractual reasons and for personal interests from those undertaken out of a sense of duty in order to promote the interests of others – allowing that financial gain is a subsidiary benefit for the professional and not a primary goal. For chaplains these characteristics should be familiar and coincide with their understanding of ministry. It is also the case, I suggest, that the idea of a responsible and professional chaplain is consistent with a vocation to serve among vulnerable and broken people in the context of health care.

Ethics in practice

Any attempt at pursuing the moral foundations of chaplaincy will repeatedly send us back to the surface where chaplaincy is practised and where, in particular encounters, the question is faced of what is the ethically right thing to do. What is the ethical response to the distraught parents in Accident and Emergency whose baby has died and who are insistent that they want their baby baptised? What is the ethical response to the young patient who confides in the chaplain that she wants to die rather than carry on with the chemotherapy? Even if we know what the ideal responses of the textbook cases are, these rarely fit with any precision the actual cases. In addition we are often deprived of the opportunity to make extensive enquiry and the time to pursue thorough reflection.

In practice, chaplains have to operate with many limitations, but this should not excuse them from acting in such a way that is able to withstand a degree of reflection and be capable of some transparency. This, according to the philosopher Bernard Williams, concerns truthfulness to self or society that cannot be answered by philosophy but 'has to be discovered, or established, as the result of a process, personal and social, which essentially cannot formulate the answer, except in an unspecific way' (1993, p.200). It is at the place of personal encounter where chaplains must live out the answers and where reasoned intentions, duties, desires, feelings and so on come into play. What ethics provides is the space for an attentive dialogue that engages with these interests and helps us to deliberate what we should do.

There are usually many interests that come into play when considering a particular situation. But this is more than a cacophony where the one who shouts loudest wins, for there are a number of voices that many consider deserve to be heard above others. Among them are those prohibiting harm, upholding freedom and calling for mutual respect. In health care, prominence is given to the distinctive voices that assert more specific rights and duties such as the vital interests of those cared for, the need for consent and the importance of holding personal information in confidence. Chaplains may also want to consider the conspicuous voices representing the moral traditions of the faith communities and, for example, the laws ecclesiastical.

All this suggests a responsible and professional approach that acknowledges substantive restrictions and requirements and locates the actions of the individual within an attentive community. Consequently, in following this process, actions are more than a subjective pursuit and they acquire a broader perspective than the individual could hope to attain. If chaplains are to maintain that they occupy public roles then this is an obligation they must attend to.

What does this all mean for the organisation and development of chaplaincy? Principally, and following the moral concerns I have high-lighted, I suggest it calls for a greater awareness of competence. Patients need to be assured that the person they are expected to trust is sufficiently skilled and knowledgeable so they may do some good and limit bad consequences. Competence is an important means of minimising the potential harm to patients inherent in many professional practices. A patient, for example, should be able to rely on a chaplain to discuss intimate matters because chaplains understand the duty of confidentiality. A nurse in intensive care dealing with a critically injured patient following a suicide attempt should be able to trust the chaplain in supporting those significant to the patient, in being sensitive to their severe emotions, and in being compassionate to their distress.

However, competence is not intended to imply a blanket guarantee for all matters dealt with; it has its limits, and a patient would be justifiably concerned about a chaplain offering physiotherapy. A characteristic of competence is that the limitations of practitioners are well understood and maintained. This has a dual benefit in that it prescribes the areas in which professionals may justifiably act whilst acknowledging the scope of their skills and expertise. Competence therefore preserves the integrity both of the professional and the patient, releasing the former from fulfilling unrealistic demands and reassuring the latter that professional boundaries will be maintained.

So the obvious question to ask is: what constitutes a competent health care chaplain? Training and education is the conventional route for a person to gain minimal professional competence that is then accompanied by the continual development of proficiency. This temporal dimension to competence is reflected typically in the career structures of professions and is alluded to in their hierarchical titles, the point being that competence for most professionals is acquired over time by gaining a body of practical knowledge and experience. In chaplaincy such a framework is somewhat aspirational and in the early stages of its development, although Martin Kerry, at Nottingham City Hospital, has implemented a competency framework (see Chapter 9). At present though, and when we look around chaplains, not even the title of 'chaplain' is a reliable indicator of a person's education, training and skills, and this is exacerbated by wide variations in job descriptions and selection criteria. There must of course be latitude within any profession and there is always going to be internal dissension and disagreement, but a reasonable degree of coherence must be a prerequisite baseline.

Competence, therefore, points to the need for an educational and professional infrastructure to ensure responsible practice and to justify public trust and finance. This means that chaplains should not be left alone in the hope that they are doing some good. In this sense it is helpful to consider chaplaincy as a discipline, even though the term has many negative connotations. A discipline implies some order, structure and direction, it suggests commitment and demands, and it indicates the outline of a *modus operandi*. To meet the ethical demands I have discussed means that the discipline is not static, introspective or opaque, but that it engages not only with the wider context in which it is practised but also with the subject it seeks to serve, aware at all times of its accountability.

The government exercises one of the most rigorous levels of accountability, and it is relevant to note in this respect the government's position on complementary and alternative medicine. Following an 18-month inquiry, the House of Lords Select Committee Report raised concerns that included a fragmented approach to self-regulation, unacceptable variations in training, lack of high-quality research, and the need for practitioners to understand the ethical aspects of health care and the nature of the therapeutic relationship (Select Committee 2000). There are clear parallels in chaplaincy, despite the obvious dissimilarities between the disciplines. Equally, there is much to be learnt from the Report including its recommendations to develop clear professional structures and regulations. Chaplaincy is not presently subject to specific public health policy, but this should not prevent it from ensuring that it can meet the ethical demands expected of those who provide patient care.

Many chaplains no doubt exercise some sort of discipline in their daily tasks, but the sort of discipline I am suggesting requires a collective dimension that is explicit in its understanding and method, fosters coherent and consistent practice and which in turn validates a distinctive identity and role. I suggest that it is this corporate aspect that is currently absent in all but a fragmented form and which will be a crucial issue if chaplaincy in Britain intends seriously to pursue state registration. It may well, of course, be the case that chaplaincy has done too little too late, and that an impatient government keen to ensure high standards across all health care disciplines will impose its own timetable.

Chaplains cannot avoid morality, even if they fail to acknowledge it as such, for their role exists primarily in relationships, and this is always a moral matter. Morality may be unavoidable for another obvious reason, and that is because it is embedded into the religious belief systems that inform both chaplains and to a greater or lesser extent the people they encounter in their work. This could be considered more problematic for health care chaplains because they are charged with providing spiritual care to a community defined by illness and injury and not by faith and culture. In other words they have to respond to the plurality of humankind that inhabit hospitals and the different moral systems they bring with them. How does a chaplain, for example, who follows the ethical stance of the Jewish tradition, respond to the fraught nurse caring for a dying Buddhist patient who has refused pain-relieving medication? How does a chaplain, who is a Muslim, respond to the young woman who follows no religion and who is in turmoil about whether to terminate her pregnancy? The obvious answer is with ethical sensitivity, which would seem to be a prerequisite for chaplaincy. But we also need to be clear that the ethical and the religious do not necessarily coincide, that moral choices can be made without a religious motivation, and that we may readily confuse a religious description of an intention with its moral quality (Holloway 1999).

If chaplaincy is to continue in its development within the NHS and justify its place in the multi-disciplinary care of patients then it is going to require a more rigorous moral base than it presently demonstrates. This may have unexpected benefits, for chaplains may discover that they are not the only ones striving to develop ethical practice, write adequate codes of conduct, and nurture accountability and competence. Chaplains may also find that other disciplines are asking interesting and important ethical questions of themselves and progressing in their ethical dialogue. What this suggests for chaplaincy is that by attending to its moral foundation it may become more self-conscious, reflective and better able to articulate its place in health care. Moreover, rather than walking on water, chaplains may find themselves walking on professional ground where the vulnerable and sacred aspect of people's lives can be entrusted to responsible and competent practitioners.

References

Dyer, C. (2000) '£1.2m for blunder that cost woman leg.' *Guardian* 31 October.

General Synod (2000) *Draft Clergy Discipline Measure 2000: GS1347A.* London: General Synod of the Church of England.

Holloway, R. (1999) *Godless Morality.* Edinburgh: Canongate.

Koehn, D. (1994) *The Ground of Professional Ethics.* London: Routledge.

Pellegrino, E. D. and Thomasma, D.C. (1997) *Helping and Healing: Religious Commitment in Health Care.* Washington D.C.: Georgetown University Press.

Porter, J. (1995) *Moral Action And Christian Ethics.* Cambridge: Cambridge University Press.

Rumbelow, H. (2000) 'Nurse tried to exorcise hospital patient.' *The Times* 5 October.

Select Committee (2000) *House of Lords Select Committee on Science and Technology Sixth Report: Complementary and Alternative Medicine.* London: The Stationery Office.

Williams, B. (1993) *Ethics and the Limits of Philosophy.* London: Fontana Press.

CHAPTER 6

Are Health Care Chaplains Professionals?

James Woodward

The world of the hospital chaplain is a complex and demanding one. As well as encountering some of the most disturbing and profound human experiences of vulnerability, illness and death, the chaplain, along with other health care workers, has to engage with the changing demands of the NHS. While some doctors and nurses still regard their career as a vocation (Whipp 1997), the chaplain remains a living symbol of the tension between vocation and career. This chapter explores one aspect of that tension – the notion of professionalism. It draws on the thought of sociologists who have attempted to define and interpret professions and discusses issues of social closure, professional dominance and managerialism in relation to health care chaplaincy.

Professions: definitions and frameworks

Sociologists have provided a range of descriptions of professions. These definitions have tended to emphasise the idea of professionals as people possessing unique skills that are put to the service of others. For many lay people the word 'professional' implies both special skills and propriety. It also implies accreditation, efficiency, competence, integrity and altruism (Pilgrim and Rogers 1993). It follows therefore that to be unprofessional is to behave incompetently, unethically, inefficiently or even fraudulently (Watson 1997).

Contemporary sociologists largely agree on the following basic propositions about characteristics of professionals:

1. Over the past two hundred years professionals have grown in influence, and expanded in both number and in types, particularly in this century.

2. Professionals provide services to people rather than produce material goods.

3. Professionals have a higher social status than manual workers through their salary or self employed status.

4. Professional status increases in relation to the length of training required to practice (doctors being an obvious example of this).

5. Professionals claim specialist knowledge about the work they do and would expect to define and control that body of knowledge.

6. Credentials give professionals a public and political credibility.

(Pilgrim and Rogers, 1993 chapter 5).

This is only a rough consensus and there is much disagreement about how professions should be understood from a sociological perspective. Durkheim, Weber, Marx and Foucault all generated frameworks for understanding professions. These, along with their relevance for chaplaincy, are outlined below.

Durkheim

For the Durkheimian tradition, professions are a source of community and stability within society. They achieve this by regulating their own practitioners and ensuring good practice through codes of conduct. Generally, professions regulate conduct in the interest of clients and to the benefit of the society they inhabit. Within this tradition the identification of a *checklist* of characteristics that distinguish professional from non-professional occupations forms the basis of a trait approach. Professionalisation is the process whereby occupations attempt to become professions by progressively acquiring these necessary characteristics. For example, the professionalisation of the clergy has seen a development in the previously haphazard approach to training programmes that integrate pastoral practice, psychology and sociology into training and ministry (Ballard and Pritchard 1998).

The relevance of the neo-Durkheimian framework to health care chaplaincy lies in the process by which chaplaincy has attempted to regulate a 'skills and outcome' approach to its work through the development of a set of occupational standards – *Health Care Chaplaincy Standards* (College of Health Care Chaplains *et al.* 1993). This established the standard of performance expected in a given work role for chaplains, offering managers a definition of competent performance in the workplace.

Weber

The Weberian tradition contains two notions relevant to this question: social closure and professional dominance. It is argued that collective professional social advancement rests upon social closure, which functions as a means of excluding occupational groups seeking similar roles. Professionals thereby restrict access to the rewards and privileges of a particular job (MacDonald 1985). Through a sharp definition of the boundaries, others are denied access and thereby kept in a state of ignorance. The maintenance of social status for professionals depends, in part, on their capacity to persuade others on the outside of their defined boundaries that they offer a unique service.

The more formal attempts by chaplains in recent years to offer a distinctive service, based on national standards and agreed outcomes, may be seen as illustrative of social closure. The attempt to establish a unique body of knowledge to underpin a new therapeutic terrain in spiritual and religious care, to the possible exclusion of others, together with their specialised activities in the area of bereavement, death and dying, staff support and education, may be interpreted as attempts to control a knowledge base which is distinctive, thereby securing their professional role and relevance in the health care institution.

The concept of professional dominance is a key feature of the Weberian understanding. This is specifically concerned with power relations. Professionals exercise power over others in three ways: they have power over clients, power over new recruits and also subordinate others within a given group. The culture of the acute hospital in particular is shaped by medical dominance, causing the chaplain to experience a marginalisation of role and identity. The setting up and development of the College of Health Care Chaplains has been part of the process of professionalisation (defining credentials, creating a distinctive knowledge base, cornering the market). From another point of view, the alliance with the MSF Union may be seen as an alternative route to the securing of some kind of professional dominance.

Marx

The Marxian tradition conceptualised power relations on the focus of vertical structural relationships. The issue for neo-Marxians is where professionals fit into a social structure which is characterised by two main groups in society: those who work to produce wealth, and those who own the means of production, exploiting the workers for profit (Larson 1977). Unsurprisingly, sociologists following a Marxian tradition of analysis have had conceptual difficulties with the professions. Professions may be deemed to be either part of the ruling class (Navarro 1979) or part of the proletariat (Oppenheimer 1975). Alternatively, they may hold a contradictory position in society, being neither capitalists, nor full members of the proletariat. Health care chaplains might be seen as being in this contradictory position: they are both agents of social control, acting on behalf of the Welfare Capitalist National Health Service, and vulnerable to the same exploitation as any other group of workers by their lack of control.

Foucault

Foucault, working within a post-structuralist framework, was interested in the relationship between knowledge and power. His framework provides a different way of looking at applied knowledge and professional work. It has no notion of a clear or stable power discrepancy between professionals and clients or between dominant professions and subordinate ones. Rather, power is dispersed and cannot be simply or easily located in any particular groupage. It is bound up with dominant, discursive features of a particular time and place, though these may be changed and resisted. For Foucault and his followers the ways in which the person – the body and mind of an individual – is described (measured, analysed and codified), are central features of contemporary society. Medicine has a central role in the surveillance of sick and healthy bodies in society.

Managerialism, dominance and closure

The introduction of general management into the NHS has had a significant impact on all health care professionals. It is clear that this change has also seriously threatened the traditional autonomy of health care chaplains. Many have been forced to become more accountable and have been made to respond to a number of challenges about the outcomes of their work in the delivery of health care. Some have secured and developed their position in the light of these challenges while others have clearly struggled to respond appropriately and creatively (Woodward 1999).

The medical profession, although similarly affected by the extension of managerial control over clinicians, has retained an unrivalled freedom to control the content of its work. The power of self-regulation and freedom from external judgement has contributed to a position of strength in relation to potential competitors, protecting medicine from boundary encroachment from other occupations. The power of medicine has in fact extended beyond self-regulation, given its monopoly over the control and organisation of health care in the wider division of labour. It has the power to direct and evaluate the work of other occupations engaged in the care of patients, without being subject to such gaze itself. The paramedical occupations, in consequence, have been excluded from the vital task of diagnosis. Their work is supervised by medicine and they lack control over their knowledge base (Larkin 1983), experiencing profound difficulties in developing their professional autonomy within health care organisations. Likewise, chaplaincy has had difficulty in defining itself as a form of paramedic group or persuading others that it is itself a therapeutic service. It has consequently remained on the margins of the debate about therapeutic intervention in the health care process.

Concluding the discussion about the sociology of professions with respect to chaplaincy, several comments can be made. It is evident that there is no agreed general definition of 'profession' when it is used by chaplains and it can be interpreted in a variety of ways. A number of debates are relevant to the development of chaplaincy. These include the process by which chaplaincy has attempted to regulate its work through the promotion of a distinctive skills, knowledge and training base. Further, it relates to the impact of the professional dominance of both managers and doctors on the culture of the NHS in general and the autonomy of chaplains in particular. The discussion about social closure is significant in respect of whether or not ordained chaplains should alone offer spiritual and religious care. This is an issue of identity and of how chaplains achieve a measure of organisational security within their hospitals. The post-structuralist framework relates to how chaplains handle the relationship between knowledge and power in their work. This discussion concerns the question of how chaplains use their theological knowledge within their work and their reflections on the context of the hospital: in other words the relationship between professional and religious identity. It is to this key theme that we now turn.

Clergy as professionals

Most sociological accounts of the clergy follow the general assumption that the clergy are a profession, to be ranked alongside lawyers, doctors, teachers and other professional groups (Parkin 1989). However, Russell (1981) argues that the apparently 'professional' developments of the clergy from the 1850s onwards have been overtaken by a new phase in which the Church begins to operate more like the voluntary societies, with fewer professionals and more part-time voluntary workers. This situation has generated an identity crisis focused on two major issues. First, whether to struggle to maintain public recognition, either by negotiation (so, health care chaplains) or by offering specialised secular skills such as counselling or therapy. The threat here is that the spiritual and religious tasks are left in the background. Second, how far to concentrate on the distinctively religious role and to work primarily with those in the churches, or else more alongside other 'caring' agencies as part of the team representing one, somewhat marginal, area of activity.

In this context the issue for health care chaplaincy is whether to accept a distinctive professional model or resist it, and if so how, in an increasingly differentiated society (Lyall 1995). It is a matter of how far the clerical role, professional as it may be in certain ways, needs even for professional purposes to retain a certain amateurism, generality and marginality. Russell lists the ways in which clergy have adopted a functionalist or trait approach to developing a professional model for themselves. There are significant difficulties in describing the clergy as a profession. These difficulties include issues of career structure, body of professional knowledge and employment practices.

Career structure

Once ordained, the clergy have no career structure. Career development (preferment) depends upon a system of organised patronage, exercised by bishops or other ecclesiastical officers but also by persons and institutions alongside the ordained ministry such as the Crown, colleges, party organisations and lay patrons.

While clergy have a strong ethos of service, a distinctive form of dress, language and folklore, and a sense of group solidarity, these are secondary professional attributes. Other occupational groups may possess these secondary characteristics but not be regarded as a profession.

Body of professional knowledge

A central concept in relation to the question of whether or not we should see the clergy as a profession relates to the assumption that theology is their body of theoretical professional knowledge. There are problematic questions over the nature and use of theology. It is not clear how much theology, as currently conveyed in the course of clergy training, is of use to health care chaplains, and how confident they are in the practical use of religious discourse in their work. Some chaplains have turned to psychotherapeutic knowledge or managerial language as a source of security for their work (Woodward 1999).

Employment practice

Finally, at present, the churches embody employment policies which discriminate against women, gays and lesbians. There are no contracts of employment with equal opportunities policies that promote an equitable framework for clergy employment. In reality, there is a tension between those who believe that the Church is a 'traditionalist' organisation and those who believe that the future is 'adaptionist' (Gill 1989). This tension has focused on the integration of women into the priesthood of the Church of England and views about the acceptability of homosexual lifestyles amongst lay and ordained Christians.

In the light of the above, two statements can be made about Anglican clergy. First, in spite of a general belief to the contrary, in many respects they are not a profession in the normal definition of the word. They may have some features characteristic of a profession but these are secondary rather than primary. In the case of health care chaplains, aspects of their adaptation to the changing context within which they work mean that they have exhibited characteristics that demonstrate aspects of professionalisation, but they cannot be regarded as a health care profession alongside other professionals in the NHS. Second, the traditional paradigm for Anglican clergy is of the single-handed parochial person. The parish continues to encapsulate several key characteristics of the Anglican clergy and is the basic unit of Anglican life. This is a significant point in relation to how health care chaplains choose to define themselves in ecclesiastical terms. If we try to think in normative terms, at best we may say that the parish is to the clergy person what the manor is to the squire: the geographical and social context in which their social status is expressed. It gives meaning to the rank conferred on a person by ordination, by ensuring there is a community that will respond to their actions, and respect their status. This is in contrast to most other professions in which the practitioner is required by clients on the functional basis of the specific service that can be provided. Specialist ministries, like health care chaplaincy, are usually undertaken by people to whom the Church gives no specialist training beforehand. They may, in addition, complain of feeling isolated and tend to define themselves in reaction or response to this parochial model, perceiving themselves to be displaced parish clergy (Legood 1998).

Towards professionalisation?

Notwithstanding the issues discussed above, there are factors which point towards the professionalisation of health care chaplains in recent years. These relate to the way pastoral carers, both within health care chaplaincy and beyond, have explored their identity and self-understanding as they work in institutional settings. In recent years, pastoral care has increasingly assumed the form of a modern profession, with the emergence of national professional societies, the promulgation of standards, the accreditation of training programmes and certification of pastoral care givers. This has generated criticism, not over the effort to ensure good quality pastoral care, but over the way these developments seems to contribute to its secularisation.

Some in chaplaincy have advocated greater professionalisation, stressing the importance of standards for the competence of pastoral carers. However, the nature of those standards has been controversial. The same role conflict we see confronting individual chaplains working between worlds exists in this collective arena where standards are being defined. Chaplains sit between the expectations of the more secular professional groups within the health care organisation on one side, and the expectations of more theologically orientated religious communities on the other. The professional groups exerting influence on the pastoral care community in this respect are primarily health care managers and central government, who have generated expectations around national frameworks and standards. The problem is that pastoral care is a religious activity and therefore its special body of knowledge, to a significant degree, is religious knowledge, itself perhaps better described as a kind of wisdom centred on spiritual practice and experience. In terms of standards, religion does not qualify as public truth but only as private belief.

Some chaplains are clearly eager to generate standards in what has previously been an ill-defined field. Chaplains are in search of an identity and degree of institutional security from whence the effects of modernisation on their role can be explored. They want their role to be understood and they want to exercise some influence on their hospitals. Inevitably, one of the challenges within the context of a professional existence is that chaplaincy is still in search of itself. This needs to be set against the feeling that retaining an element of amateurishness is part of the chaplain's usefulness. In contrast, the process of hospitalisation and the structures which control the delivery, tasks and functions of health care are very clearly defined. This is a regimented structure with clearly defined boundaries both between and within professions.

Unsurprisingly, the question of how the chaplain fits in to this clearly demarcated process is both challenging and problematical. The institutional position of the chaplain is not a neat one, and in order to perform the functions and tasks of pastoral care within the hospital a number of tools will be needed. These include anthropology, psychology and management skills as well as the normal ministerial training in theology and pastoral care. A whole range of factors will bear upon meanings of illness in a hospital and the chaplain is required to be flexible in both thinking and practice. The hospital acts as a kind of threshold that transforms a number of traditions and produces its own world of religious meanings, if largely divorced from the world of the Church. This hospital world is attractive and energising for some chaplains; for others it is complex, devaluing and confusing.

Despite the growth in numbers of chaplains and some measure of increase in professional competency, hospital chaplains remain in some ways an enigma to themselves, the churches and the health care world. What is clear is that the success of health care chaplaincy lies in the personal characteristics of the individual chaplain. Chaplains define their personal identity individually rather than through a tradition or corporate identity such as the College of Health Care Chaplains. They are often admired as men and women; sometimes as acceptable faces of religion and at other times as people who have listened and supported with a huge amount of sensitivity and skill. It follows then that while the role and functions of the chaplain may be enigmatic, their personal characteristics are not. Chaplains are appreciated for their personal warmth, approachability and readiness to support staff. These characteristics are both valued and affirmed.

Perhaps this hints at the dangers in the adoption of professionalisation strategies. It may not be desirable to define too closely the art of hospital chaplaincy. It is a ministry of dialogue and of the exchange of ideas and feelings. It is always on the move; always changing, partial, informal and always passing by and through. Its constant feature, in addition to the strength of the personal characteristics of the chaplain, is the readiness and skill in listening to the voices of suffering. This is the unique function of the hospital chaplain, which some understand and value and others mistrust. In embracing a philosophy of the human ecology – that is the understanding and care of human beings as whole persons in the light of their relationships to God, to themselves, their families and a society in which they live – the chaplain continues to be a resource for the processes by which we live with our suffering. Chaplains therefore find themselves easily enmeshed in conflict. Their role is not to explain, cure or eliminate disease. It is to engage with the sufferer in the suffering, and to embrace it with sensitive pastoral care.

At the heart of ministry lies a conviction about the nature and person of God. A minister is a vocational professional in the sense that one of the undergirding questions motivating his or her work is: 'what does God want of me?' It is important, therefore, to ask how theology might become a useful tool in the attempt to move the ministry of the health care chaplain to an acceptable professional base within the health service. Perhaps in a desire for security, the chaplain prefers to adopt and appropriate many of the cultural norms prevalent within the organisation of health care itself?

It is within the context of the hospital as a secular institution that the Christian chaplain has to work out his or her obedience to the gospel. There is a theological basis for working with the culture as 'given' by the creator. There is a need to state a belief in God as not confined to the religious sphere or embattled against non-Christian structures, but as involved in all parts of creation. It is in this context that the need to be professional and the negotiation of freedom in controlling the content of chaplaincy work seem to be significant, but there are certain dangers in the ethos of professionalism. There may be some uncertainty or confusion about what 'professional' means in this discussion. For chaplains it is partly to do with being efficient and co-operative in relation to the hospital structures, and this understanding is to be encouraged; but it cannot stand alone. The issue is in part about a chaplain's sense of identity and role within the hospital. There will, of course, be some chaplains who hold the structures and value systems at arm's length while they continue their activity. This approach is, I believe, defective.

Health care chaplaincy has no option but to organise and develop a professional approach to its key tasks, but there are dangers. The organisation of health care is often ambiguous and complex. There is a need to get the chaplains' feet under the organisational table but often to remain on the edges and margins, and risk feeling impotent as a result. In the light of this, refuge may be taken in clear roles in order to cope with the feelings of insecurity: the chaplain as academic; the chaplain as manager; the chaplain as therapist. Perhaps a chaplain needs to be critically reflective about where self-validation comes from. It will not necessarily come from the attempt to be professional in a narrow sense. In the debate about clarity of roles and tasks, what part is there for the intangible, the immeasurable and the transcendent?

One of the areas within which there is a major theological crisis is in the chaplain's critique of the culture of which he or she is a part. Chaplains seem reluctant to take on the role of saboteur, mole or whistle blower. More reflection needs to be done on the assumption of the implicit goodness of the organisation and culture of health care today. In this sense chaplains have understandably become institutionalised. Their loyalty is with the hospital that pays them. There is discomfort in asking 'with whom or to whom do chaplains need to belong?' The role of the prophet is an almost impossible one to fulfil when the chaplain depends upon the hospital for validation and security.

In a postmodern world, clergy are not absent. They may be mis-understood but they still stand as valid representative figures. In the health service, chaplains live with paradox and tension; engaging with marginal-isation and disempowerment. They are present in and potential transformers of the experience of illness in relation to staff, patients and their families and friends. It is perhaps inevitable that chaplains are odd, but maybe this is where their strength lies: not in their professionalisation but in their liminality. Their marginal position allows them to listen, to interpret and to share meanings and activities which in essence are liberating and trans-forming. Hospitals may well be poorer places without them.

References

Ballard, P. and Pritchard, J. (1998) *Practical Theology in Action: Christian Thinking in the Service of Church and Society.* London: SPCK.

College of Health Care Chaplains, Free Church Hospital Chaplaincy Board, Hospital Chaplaincies Council, Roman Catholic Hospital Chaplaincies (1993) *Health Care Chaplaincy Standards.* Bristol: NHS Training Directorate.

Gill, R. (1989) *Competing Convictions*. London: SCM Press.

Larkin, G. V. (1983) *Occupational Monopoly and Medicine*. London: Tavistock.

Larson, M. S. (1977) *The Rise of Professionalism*. California: University of California Press.

Legood, G. (1998) *Chaplaincy: The Church's Sector Ministries*. London: Cassell.

Lyall, D. (1995) *Counselling in the Pastoral and Spiritual Context*. Buckingham: Open University Press.

MacDonald, K. M. (1985) 'Social closure and occupational registration.' *Sociology 19*, 4, 541–556.

Navarro, V. (1979) *Medicine Under Capitalism*. New York: Prodist.

Oppenheimer, M. (1975) 'The proletarianisation of the professional.' *Sociological Review*, Monograph, 20.

Parkin, F. (1989) *Max Weber*. London: Routledge.

Pilgrim, D. and Rogers, A. (1993) *A Sociology of Mental Health and Illness*. Buckingham: Open University Press.

Russell, A. (1981) *The Clerical Profession*. London: SPCK.

Watson, T. (1997) *Sociology Work and Industry*. London: Routledge.

Whipp, M. (1997) 'A Healthy Sense of Vocation?' *Contact 122*, 3–10.

Woodward, J. (1999) 'A Study of the Role of the Acute Health Care Chaplain in England.' Unpublished PhD thesis of the Open University.

CHAPTER 7

Speaking of the Same Things Differently

Christopher Swift

All seeing is perspectival. There is no neutral vantage point and no totalising vision. (Prosser MacDonald 1995, p.37)

In the spring of 1998 I presented a paper on chaplaincy to the Executive Directors' Group of the hospital where I am chaplain. Having listened to it, the Chief Executive reflected that hearing me talk about the hospital was to hear 'the same things spoken about differently'. It was a straightforward yet profound remark that hinted at the relationships between location, patterns of working and the nature of observation. We shared the same space, but saw things in different ways – and invested that seeing with a variety of meanings. This chapter will attempt to explore some of this diversity. It will go on to describe ways in which postmodern writers offer models of enquiry to chaplains that might assist them in a deeper understanding of the complex organisations in which they work. And, although the focus will be on chaplaincy, it has implications for all those concerned for spiritual care in health.

Chaplains currently stand in a fascinating place. Formed by cultures derived from their faith communities they are regarded by colleagues as religious leaders (clergy, imams and so on), while at the same time being fully absorbed into the employment structures of the NHS. It is also a position still widely open to individual interpretation, with few formal guidelines for the day-to-day practice of chaplaincy. Some use detailed forms of spiritual assessment, others the most informal and unrecorded kinds of encounter. This ambiguous position and disparity of practice is set within a culture of national standards and regular audit for other disciplines involved in health care. Chaplaincy sometimes is, and quite often isn't, included in a variety of key arrangements that apply to other disciplines. Its diffuse central structures, rooted in faith communities and denominations, illustrate the odd relationship that it has within the NHS.

How chaplaincy has arrived at this position is an interesting subject in itself – and one as yet unaddressed. Chaplains were the chief element in the central structures of medieval and post-Reformation hospitals. Even in Victorian times they held substantial sway in hospitals, as well as in the growing number of workhouses with their fledgling infirmaries. The observation that in this later period the chaplain was the 'Sunday gaoler' (Crowther 1983, p.128) indicates that their role could be described as having a disciplinary function. With the establishment of the NHS, the place of chaplains began to alter and, set in the context of wider changes in Church and society, their role seems to be increasingly marginal and open to question. Such a situation might be uncomfortable for some chaplains, but it is not necessarily fruitless.

I want to suggest that the peculiar combination of features which position chaplaincy within the NHS today give it unique vantage. This is not to claim that chaplaincy somehow holds the 'key' to understanding health care, or that its view is privileged over the perspective of others. Yet it does imply that something valuable could be lost if the general position of chaplaincy was to shift. As the College of Health Care Chaplains explores the possibility of state registration, spiritual care givers need to reflect on their position with both imagination and insight. In what follows I will set out some examples of the observations chaplains make, and how these might be understood in postmodern terms. The chapter concludes with some consideration of what might be done with these insights – and how they in turn question the role of spiritual care givers.

Hearing differently

There are many postmodern thinkers who would question the idea that there are things within any organisation that could be described as 'the same'. These commentators would suggest instead that what we see in a health care setting arises out of the discourses that are created by individuals and groups (Morris 1998, pp.21f). In other words, we can never directly know a *thing* – its existence is always alluded to in discourse but never fully captured by it. Language washes over our surroundings, is channelled into stronger currents here and weaker ones there, but never ceases to be fluid. How language is constructed, directed and discharged therefore forms the basis upon which writers such as Foucault explore the role of professions in their address to the body (Foucault 1979). The regulation of the body is the crucial element of a postmodern critique that challenges the role of those engaged in all aspects of health care.

In terms of NHS management, Stephen Pattison has explored the implicit values and beliefs that drive the current form of the profession. He observes that theories of management contain 'basic moral values and practices which shape a vision of the world and what it is to be human' (Pattison 1997, p.5). These powerful claims about the beliefs of a modern profession are equally suitable for examining the values and practices of others involved in the NHS. From a Foucaultian perspective the way to do this is by examining what happens to the sick body, questioning how it is received, handled and interrogated. How, in other words, the perceived fact of the body enters into discourse.

Questions that this approach might formulate run something like this: in what ways does the discourse within a health care setting construct the body?; what language surrounds the body, how is it defined and organised by those who address it? Let me take a simple illustration of this, and one familiar to all those working in hospitals:

Chaplain:	How are you doing Mrs A?
Mrs A:	Not so bad, but they say I can't go home this week.

This short and typical exchange demonstrates one way in which discourse frames the patient. By coming into hospital we are not co-workers in our own health, but the objects of medical discipline. The exchange cited above could have run like this:

Chaplain:	How are you doing Mrs B?
Mrs B:	Not so bad, the doctor doesn't think I am well enough to go home this week – I've thought about it, and I'm going to take his advice.

But it hardly ever does. In this first case Mrs A is the passive recipient of medical inscription. She has been told that her body is too dysfunctional to be discharged. There is no contestation of this view, and she waits for new measurements of progress to be taken – new inspections of her body – which need to be satisfied before she will be permitted to go home. In the second case Mrs B implies that the choice of discharge is her own – that she makes the decisions about her body – and that the role of medicine is to advise her in that decision. Only in the second example is there the sense that medical knowledge is accountable to the patient and not, as in the first case, the other way round.

.The key point here is that attention to language in health care settings begins to reveal some of the implicit workings of power within an organisation. The fact of what is said should not be neglected or brushed aside by the assumption that the patient *really* means x, y or z. Because the concept of what people really mean, despite what they say, is one of the most fundamental attributes of disciplinary power. Its operation serves the interest of professionalism – often under the guise of being good for the patient – in such a way that individual experience is bound to correspond to patterns already deemed acceptable. To resist such inscription is a painful and sometimes costly act.

In the context of the NHS the body is often understood as individual, ideally passive, and open to the inscription of medical and institutional meaning. Most of us who use it appear to make an unspoken transaction in which responsibility for our bodies is given up in exchange for professional care. Foucault has noted many of the characteristics of professional power, not least the use of a language peculiar to the discipline; the observation and categorisation of the body; the growth of technologies to turn knowledge into physical action (Foucault 1980). Above all else it is vital that professional knowledge is beyond immediate public question. Its enquiries into the physical world aim at conclusions that are attainable, instrumental and universal.

By comparison, spiritual knowledge is widely held in the NHS to be a matter of personal expertise, in which the care giver assists the patient in their own 'treatment'. For Christian chaplains the principal texts of their profession sit in the patient's locker. This availability is made, irrespective of whether or not the patient has achieved some recognised level of comp- rehension. The interaction of patient and religious text is a fundamentally open one, with perhaps only a few indications at the front as to what passages might match up with certain experiences. What the existence of these texts illustrate (whether patients use them or not) is that Christian patients have the implied authority to take a valid view of their spiritual care. There may be denominational/faith differences about how the role of a priest/minister/scholar mediates elements of the text – but the fact of the text is on the patient's side in many traditions.

Other professions might see this as a sign of weakness – the purchase of groups within the NHS depending upon the possession of knowledge unattained by others. The role of spiritual care givers is to provide a relationship with patients within the context of the patient's own spiritual traditions. At the patient's request – or in response to an offer made to them – certain rites may be enacted at the bedside. But the patient's choice about the appropriateness of these remains paramount.

While the chaplain may possess a deeper knowledge and experience in the meta-narrative of their faith, this is not generally regarded as a pretext for religious inscription within a hospital. Let me illustrate this point with a hypothetical – and *perhaps* extreme – scenario:

> The Senior Chaplain enters the ward at a brisk pace, accompanied by a group of his assistants. Approaching Mrs Jones he exchanges a brief smile before peering over his glasses at the notes he is carrying.
>
> 'Now Mrs Jones, Dr Mitchell has asked me to come along and see you. How are you doing?' Mrs Jones looks apprehensive and mutters something that sounds like 'not so bad' – then quickly looks at the small group assembled around her.
>
> 'Well, Dr Mitchell felt that you were having some concerns about the *meaning* of what is happening to you. Is that right?' Mrs Jones nods cautiously.
>
> 'Now', (he peers at the notes again) 'it appears that you've been having Methodism for quite some time'.
>
> 'Yes, on and off for about 60 years. But it all seems rather pointless now.'
>
> 'Mmm, let me see. Well I think you may be suffering from something we call "Dark Night of the Soul". I wouldn't be too worried if I were you. There has been a lot of research recently in cases like yours, and I think we might be able to help. We're going to try you on something a little more *Catholic* for a few days. Does that sound all right?'
>
> Without pausing for an answer the Senior Chaplain busily writes out a prescription. Turning to a junior he hands over the script. 'Make sure she says these prayers morning

and evening until Thursday – and I've also prescribed a short course of Bible readings. OK?'

The Senior Chaplain smiles weakly at Mrs Jones, and walks off smartly to see another patient – the troop of juniors chasing after him.

Spiritual care givers do not work like this (although I have met one or two chaplains who might like to!) And if this excessively medical illustration seems not to be a model for chaplaincy, I do not believe that disciplines such as clinical psychology offer better examples. The small basis of mutual expectation that exists between a C of E chaplain and a Christian patient (in some sense or other, we are both Christians) is missing in the encounter with the therapist. What does the psychologist believe, what are her values? As with other professions these questions are not seen to be relevant – only practitioners need to know the theories of human growth and change on which their work rests. However, the idea that any psychological work is 'value free' is a potentially self-deluding notion (Goodliff 1998, pp.86f). Nikolas Rose's *Governing the Soul* (1999) is the clearest exploration of how these technologies of the self have been employed to extend the boundaries of disciplinary power. This new approach to the subject works to internalise surveillance – enlisting us as co-workers in a psycho-medical project controlled by professional authority.

One possible approach for spiritual care givers that resists the disposition to classify patient experience could be described as 'attentive waiting'. The chaplain is not the expert in the patient's spiritual state – she must wait on the patient, and strive to give open attention. It is a largely unbounded attitude that brings with it little intention to 'do' for the patient but a determined effort to 'be' for them. Commenting on the work of Maurice Blanchot, Zigmunt Bauman writes:

> Such an attention, such *waiting*, is not possessive; it does not aim at dispossessing the Other of her will, of her distinctiveness and identity – through physical coercion, or the intellectual conquest called 'the definition'. (1993, p.88)

Of course this has by no means been the chief characteristic of traditional spiritual care. 'Pastoral power' is a target for a great deal of criticism by Foucault and others – largely because its coercion passes for a virtue that can generate both guilt and gratitude (Bauman 1993, p.103). But the re-definition of spirituality in health care (a matter of personal choice; a plurality of possible responses shaped by traditions and relationships) has opened the way for a new attitude of attention and waiting. Sufficiently unconstricted by the clinical patterns of formal care, the person addressing spiritual needs has the potential to offer their presence as 'gift'. Nick Fox's work in this area will strike many familiar chords with chaplains and other workers concerned with spiritual care. Unlike the disciplines which aim to 'help' the patient to pre-conceived ends, the gift-meeting is an encounter 'constituted in an open-endedness' (Fox 1993, p.102). It generates difference and possibility without limiting those to the requirements of audit and protocols. Most importantly, it does not define the discourse it hears – it does not locate it in a hierarchy of pre-established significance.

It follows that one of the difficult questions for spiritual care givers is how their approach can find value in a setting overwhelmingly committed to a largely instrumental attitude to research and evidence. Many chaplains believe that their unique vantage and ambiguous status generates encounters that are difficult to fit into the criteria of other disciplines – yet are nevertheless valuable within health care. Perhaps chaplaincy needs to develop a new question – a new way of assessing value in the NHS. If a manager were to ask me why there should be chaplains I would probably reply by telling a story. Because story is precisely that subjective and particular kind of discourse which illustrates the patient–chaplain encounter in ways statistics (of whatever sort) never can (Macnaughton 1995). It may be that spiritual care givers need to adopt qualitative research techniques that present story in a way intelligible for the NHS.

Acting differently

Chaplaincy could go down the road of benchmarking its assistance to patients; of targeting levels of acceptable progress; of creating classifications for 'spiritual health'. But, as I have indicated above, there is a price to pay for this apparent clarity. The satisfaction of criteria defined at a distance from the patient – certainly the patient in front of you *now* – can limit the recognition of individual need. 'Pathways' and 'protocols' serve a purpose, but what of the patient whose experience strays from the norm: do we change our path or change theirs?

Can things be different for spiritual care givers in general, and chaplains in particular? If chaplaincy wants to choose its future direction then it has some obligation to reflect on the possible models set out before it. Foucault's approach to the historic rise of disciplinary power, and what he calls 'the history of the present', requires close attention to the technologies of care (Dean 1994, p.21). Those engaged in addressing spiritual issues need to reflect on their daily pattern of work, their conversation and their movement through the environment of care. At one level it is as important and as simple as asking which doors you can walk through and the kinds of people it is possible to speak with. It is a reflective practice that begins to disclose the nature of power and its boundaries. The value of this exercise is that *disclosed* techniques of power become more problematic to utilise, and disciplinary power is driven to reinvent itself.

To illustrate this I give what may seem a trivial example, but nevertheless one which demonstrates the possibility of challenge. At a multi-disciplinary meeting concerning a group of patients the consultant was struggling to recall someone's condition. 'Oh, she's a…she's a…'. I couldn't resist, and supplied him with the word 'Baptist'. In a shorthand world of medical inscription defended by the need for efficiency patients are literally defined by their disease. It is not the language of they *have*, but the ontological statement that they *are*. At an individual level there is perhaps little that a chaplain can do other than to draw attention to this way of talking, and thereby question its underlying assumptions. But if the vantage of the chaplain makes it possible to question the culture of talking about patients in the way I have described, is there not a responsibility to articulate those concerns more widely? Is there a way for spiritual care givers to facilitate discussion of concerns about the nature of the medical gaze that is exercised by many working in the NHS?

Let me take one further illustration. A hospital has a discrepancy between the expected uptake of Halal food and the number of patients likely to request it. In fact a lot of food appears to be brought in by families – disrupting the hospital's ability to control and manage the patient diet. What questions does the hospital ask itself? Is the communication being done effectively? Are staff recording requests accurately? Is it being served properly? Is the food up to a sufficient standard? Given its preoccupations with care plans and the clinical aspects of diet it does not ask itself 'What is food – what does it mean to take a meal?' In many Muslim households it is a form of worship, and a way in which individuals are included in family life. The peculiar place of chaplaincy can incline it to question the nature of the assumptions being made – and to challenge the scope of permissible meanings. But it will do this with greater success if it can work to sensitise others to the issues involved.

Chaplaincy may need to re-value its current role, and gain a greater confidence in its ability to speak out to other elements within the health care setting. I want to suggest that it has valuable attributes that could lead it to the revision of some of its current practices and possibly to develop new ones. Most significantly from this perspective, chaplaincy offers a unique space for the expression of *indefinite hope* within the medical environment. This hope is characterised by its inability to fit neatly into established systems (it is often ambiguous) as well as by its qualities of persistence. The gift that spiritual care can offer to those articulating indefinite hope is an openness for such expressions to stand as they are – and not to be re-invented by a body of disciplinary knowledge. As a patient once put it to me: 'I can talk to you because you don't write everything down – you don't put a label on what I'm telling you'.

Chaplains, and those who share in spirituality within hospitals, have the gift of possibilities that are excluded elsewhere. Let me develop this further with the common sight of a prayer board in the hospital chapel. This small surface is the only space given for the inscription by patients, relatives and staff of hopes that in other contexts would be deemed irrational and discounted – for recovery in the face of the body's apparently total failure; for reunion with those who have died; for blessing on a life cursed with all kinds of breakdown. These prayers are not the response to a question, but to a space able to resonate with the absences that people experience. And what is written on prayer boards is replicated in spoken or silent prayer in the chapel or prayer room and in bedside conversations with chaplains. What spiritual care givers offer – and should be loath to lose – is a spaciousness for those who may find their hopes all too often enmeshed in medical meaning.

New trajectories

The work of chaplains could be to remain open to such articulations of hope – of defiance of the boundaries dictated by disciplinary power. Such a direction for the work of spiritual care givers necessitates an active and reflective engagement with the discourses of power – not least pastoral power. At a crucial time in their profession health care chaplains need to weigh up the trajectories that might emerge in the wider world of the NHS. Spiritual and pastoral involvement offers some interesting possibilities to those who manage care, including the reconciliation of patients to the processes of health. But do chaplains want – or believe it is right – to become the spiritual acolytes of medical or managerial power (Nelson 1992, p.131)?

Spiritual care givers are already aware that their involvement with patients can be triggered by the inability of a ward to cope with or pacify their client. A professionalisation modelled on other health care disciplines could enhance chaplaincy status – but at what price for both patient and chaplain?

I have attempted to describe how chaplaincy offers something unique within the health care setting – that it can both hear and speak differently. The presence of a professional group at the periphery of many areas of hospital life – yet plunged into the centre on occasions – adds a value to the insights of the organisation that would be difficult to achieve elsewhere. The questions that chaplains can ask, and the people to whom they can address them, illustrate a view often obscured in the rest of health care. 'What *is* food?', '*Why* is a patient what they suffer?', are reflections into the heart of hospital life, thrown from the margins of medical power. Of course it may be the case that those to whom such questions are addressed themselves feel trapped by practices that prohibit any serious engagement with these ideas. It is this experience that provides opportunity for the articulation of 'indefinite hope' – of having someone to speak with who sits ambiguously yet openly in the environment of clinical truth.

The future crisis for the traditional givers of spiritual care lies in the increasing tension between the worlds to which chaplaincy belongs. In particular the growing regulation and governance of practices within the NHS require a greater definition of the chaplain's spiritual role. At the same time, state registration seems an inevitable path if chaplains wish to remain as a professional body in health care. How that process unfolds, and with what consequences for chaplains and those they serve, remains to be seen. All spiritual care givers need to reflect on the integrity of what they offer – and how such care is used within the powerful discourses of health. The responsibilities for chaplains to think about what they do and where they work seem inherent in the beliefs of a number of the faith traditions from which they come. Believing that the spiritual dynamics of the NHS are implicitly good does not make them so – chaplains owe greater insight to a calling than that. If spiritual care givers want to reflect like this then ways of doing so need to be constructed. One avenue might be through a greater involvement for chaplains in the statements on social responsibility made by their faith or denomination.

The poet Philip Larkin was once asked how he managed to write such perceptive and well-crafted verse. He replied that he simply wrote down what he saw. The key to that remark lies in the place of the observer and their capacity to describe what they see. I believe that the peculiar constitution of chaplains invites them to look at the hospital environment differently. To question its meanings – its implicit construction of patients and staff – and to speak and act in new ways. In this they are able to give a spaciousness to the expression of spirituality which is a unique and vital element for those caught up in the powerful dynamics of health care. Chaplaincy is a presence that has the capacity to hear the indefinite hope of those in hospital – and not to turn that hope into its own meaning.

References

Bauman, Z. (1993) *Postmodern Ethics*. Oxford: Blackwell.

Crowther, M. A. (1983) *The Workhouse System, 1834–1929: The History of an English Social Institution*. London: Methuen.

Dean, M. (1994) *Critical and Effective Histories*. London: Routledge.

Foucault, M. (1979) *Discipline and Punish*. London: Penguin Books.

Foucault, M. (1980) *Power/Knowledge*. Harlow, Essex: Harvester Press.

Fox, N. (1993) *Beyond Health*. London: Free Association Books.

Goodliff, P. (1998) *Care in a Confused Climate*. London: Darton, Longman and Todd.

Macnaughton, J. (1995) 'Anecdotes and empiricism.' *British Journal of General Practice*, November, 571–572.

Morris, D. B. (1998) *Illness and Culture*. California: University of California Press.

Nelson, J. B. (1992) *Body Theology*. Louisville: Westminster/John Knox Press.

Pattison, S. (1997) *The Faith of the Managers*. London: Cassell.

Prosser MacDonald, D. L. (1995) *Transgressive Corporeality*. New York: State University of New York Press.

Rose, N. (1999) *Governing the Soul*. 2nd edn; London: Free Association Books.

CHAPTER 8

Spiritual Crisis? Call a Nurse

Wilfred McSherry

Introduction

It could be argued that nurses are the rightful custodians of all matters spiritual. It would appear that from a historical perspective this 'order' or duty was bequeathed and conferred because of the unique position they held and still hold in the delivery of health care. Their presence and professionalism graces and supports individual patients, their families and indeed all who are sick, diseased, vulnerable, dying and in constant need throughout the 24-hour day.

However, to many professionals working in today's 'Modern and Dependable' National Health Service, this statement may seem presumptuous, bold, unfounded and perhaps naive. This position seems untenable and indeed unjustified at a time when health care is experiencing change and reforms, calling for greater accountability through inter-disciplinary collaboration. However, emerging research suggests nurses do perceive themselves to be key stakeholders in the spiritual dimension of care as they attempt to address and implement the rhetoric of holism; that is, caring for all quarters of the individual: physical, psychological, social and spiritual (Griffin 1993; Ham-Ying 1993).

There is a growing realisation within health care and increasingly by nurses, that there is a fundamental need to attend to the spiritual needs of their patients. The exact reasons for this may in part be explained by dissatisfaction with the scientific and managerial models that have guided medical and to some extent nursing practice. This growing awareness is also echoed in recent times by the drive to have spirituality formally integrated within programmes of nurse education. However, the result of such innovations may end in a blurring of boundaries between all professional groups involved in the provision of spiritual care. The net effect may be that spiritual care becomes fragmented or hindered and lost in dispute over issues of role and responsibility. This chapter will explore these issues in further detail, concluding with a call for multi-disciplinary collaboration in all matters spiritual.

Historical perspectives

It is recognised that nursing and indeed health care has a rich spiritual heritage (Swaffield 1988; Bradshaw 1996). Tracing the historical development of nursing reveals that it originated from religious and monastic communities (Carson 1989; Narayanasamy 1999). These communities of priests, monks and brothers sanctified their own souls in works of mercy by sacrificing themselves through caring for the sick, dying and destitute. There was a realisation that to 'care' meant not only treating the physical. These communities recognised the relationship and intricate balance between mind, body, and spirit. As they strove to give witness to the Christian 'Beatitudes' (Matt. 5) they ministered to the sick, both physically and spiritually. It is suggested that the spiritual took precedence over the physical in the priority of care. Caring and ultimately nursing evolved out of this time of spiritual enlightenment.

The spiritual was not divorced, or viewed in isolation, from other dimensions of the person. It seemed the spiritual dimension, founded on religious principles, was at the centre of their philosophies and theories of care. This sentiment is shared by Narayanasamy who writes: 'In earlier times the distinction between medicine and nursing was not clear but from the middle ages onwards nursing evolved as a distinct profession through the influence of spirituality.' (Narayanasamy 1999, p.394)

This holistic approach remained central and fundamental to the notion of nursing. It could be argued that this was the case until the 19th century. Up until this point, religious orders of nuns were primarily responsible for providing care. However, there followed a 'u-turn' as they lost their position in a radically changing society. The state began to assert its authority, becoming more active and interested in concerns of a welfare nature (Carson 1989; Narayanasamy 1999). It could be argued that this political involvement threatened the position of religious communities who were nursing the sick and caring for the destitute.

Erosion of the spiritual

McSherry (2000) argues that the reform and advance of medical science in the 20th century resulted in the infiltration of a scientific model that eroded the spiritual heritage of nursing. The hard, concrete face of science has replaced nursing's spiritual heritage. Of course, not all scientific and medical advancements have had a negative effect – some have increased longevity, rid the world of disease and provided hope for many in the future. Nevertheless, some schools of thought argue that medical science has brought new moral and ethical dilemmas in matters concerning the sanctity of life, especially in the field of embryology.

Refocusing upon the spiritual

More recently, the general public has called for the medical profession to re-evaluate its image because of a dissatisfaction with a purely medical approach to care. As a result of such dissatisfaction some health care professions have reinvested energy and interest in the spiritual dimension. This is evident in the vast number of books, articles and research studies appearing on the subject (Narayanasamy 1991; Harrison and Burnard 1993; Bradshaw 1994; Farmer 1996; Ross 1997; Cobb and Robshaw 1998; McSherry 2000). It would appear that there is a growing realisation that science does not possess all the answers to some of the profound existential questions raised by patients (Harrison 1993). This re-focusing upon the importance of spirituality within health care (and specifically in nursing) indicates a change of opinion, presenting a major challenge to the scientific community. With respect to matters of spirituality, patients (and indeed other health care professions) are turning to nursing to show them the way. The question and answer posed in the title of this chapter: 'Spiritual crisis? Call a nurse' may well be justified; although it warrants further explanation.

The frontline

Nurses hold a unique position in the delivery of patient care. They are present 24 hours a day, 7 days a week, 365 days a year. This continual presence places them at the centre of care delivery (Stoter 1995). Because of this position they are more likely to be the first to encounter a patient presenting with a spiritual need. Contemporary research confirms that nurses of all grades are identifying patients with spiritual need (Waugh 1992; McSherry 1997).

This interest in the spiritual dimension within nursing is not confined to 'general' or palliative care settings but across all branches of nursing: adult, paediatric (Kenny 1999), learning disability (Birchenall 1987; Males and Boswell 1990; Balkizas and O'Hare 1994) and mental health (Mickley, Carson and Soeken 1995). Pioneering research conducted in the USA from the 1970s onwards (and latterly in the UK) has resulted in a steady flow of research, generating debate about the conceptual and theoretical construct of spirituality (Cawley 1997). More importantly, there is a growing discussion about the relevance of such theories to clinical practice (Oldnall 1995). Nurses are acutely aware that if justice is to be done in this dimension of care it cannot remain a theoretical construct but must be implemented and applied in practice.

Nursing the spirit

The spiritual needs of an individual are not left at the entrance to the hospital or care setting. For some patients, illness or hospitalisation may actually result in a re-focusing or questioning of their spirituality (Murray and Zentner 1989). An illness, or indeed any crisis, may act as a trigger which moves the individual to revisit, encounter or 'get in touch with' their own spirituality (Narayanasamy 1996). McSherry (2000) suggests that, at some point during the course of their working practice, nurses will find that a patient under their care has a spiritual need.

Recent research undertaken by nurses reveals they see the importance of attending to the spiritual needs of patients (Waugh 1992; Narayanasamy 1993; McSherry 1997). There seems to be a realisation by nurses that attending to this aspect of care is synonymous with issues surrounding quality of life and a person's well-being (Ross 1995). This is not to suggest that all nurses are confident and comfortable in attending to patients' spiritual needs – in fact the reverse has been shown (Narayanasamy 1993; McSherry 1997). Johnston, Taylor, Highfield and Amenta highlight this unease, commenting: '...nurses' commitment to, or confidence about, spiritual care is not as strong as could be' (Johnston et al. 1994, p.485). Nevertheless, emerging research indicates that nurses have a willingness to be involved in delivering spiritual care and have expressed a desire to gain a deeper understanding about the subject. It could be argued that these two aptitudes – *willingness* and *desire for new knowledge* – are a sure foundation on which to develop future education and practice.

A systematic approach

The central position nurses hold in the delivery of health care means that they are often with patients throughout their entire period of hospital-isation. They are usually involved in every stage; from admission right through to discharge. Ensuring that the care provided is effective and efficient requires careful planning and consideration. To assist in the process of care delivery, nurses have been using a reliable and valid framework for several years, known as 'The Nursing Process'. This states:

> The nursing process is a problem-solving approach to nursing that involves interaction with the patient, making decisions and carrying out nursing actions based on an assessment of an individual patient's situation. It is followed by an evaluation of the effectiveness of our actions. (Kratz 1979, p.3)

The nursing process can assist in the delivery of nursing care that is individualised and patient-centred – that involves the patient in the entire process. Care is not planned in isolation or without consultation. The nursing process enables nurses to assess, plan, implement and evaluate their interventions. This systematic approach can be applied to patients who may present with a spiritual need (Ross 1996).

Spiritual assessment

The notion of spiritual assessment is gaining momentum in health care (Stoll 1979; Catteral *et al.* 1998; Cobb 1998; McSherry 2000). However, caution should be exercised as the area is not as straightforward as it may first appear. There are many ways in which an assessment of spiritual need could be conceived and numerous methods available (such as continuous assessment, direct questioning or measurement scales). From the author's experience, there appears to be a drive to create an assessment tool that can be used universally within a hospital Trust. Such assessment tools are designed to be quick and simple – probably producing some quantitative measure of need. A danger in constructing and using such tools is that they will reduce the assessment of spirituality to a mechanistic or 'tick box' exercise (McSherry 2000), devaluing other modes of assessment that health care professionals use. The term 'assess*ment*' is itself problematic, sometimes being understood as an activity which is carried out only once. Perhaps the term 'assess*ing*' would be more appropriate in the context of spirituality, indicating a need for continual surveillance and vigilance by all health care professionals.

During the course of admitting a patient into their ward or under their care, nurses may ask specific questions related to the patient's activities of living. Most admission documents will contain a section that enables the nurse to inquire about a patient's religious affiliation or beliefs and there may even be a section termed '*spiritual needs*'. The author's own experience in using such documentation indicates that nurses and indeed patients sometimes have difficulty in knowing what to ask, write or say. Audits of nursing records reveal that it is not uncommon to find this section left blank or containing simply the abbreviation 'C of E', with no further indication of the extent of an individual's religious practices. This is concerning as it suggests patients' religious and spiritual needs may not be adequately assessed by nurses upon admission to a health care setting. The practice also contradicts the expectations of *The Patient's Charter* (DoH 1996).

Nevertheless, it is clear nurses have a key role to play in the identification of patients who may present with a spiritual need during a period of hospitalisation (Simsen 1985). This role is one of duty: nurses' professional practice is guided by statutory and professional expectations. Yet one would hope a nurse, by using a range of assessment methods and by developing a plan of care in collaboration with the patient, would be able to assist patients in meeting their spiritual needs. This is a gross over-simplification because there are many barriers that may inhibit this relationship, preventing the nurse from enabling the patient to achieve a particular goal or spiritual need. However, before the nursing profession is blamed for failing to provide adequate spiritual care, an exploration of possible reasons for this is required.

Barriers

There is still a great deal of misconception and ambiguity surrounding the term 'spirituality'. This can result in the formation of barriers or defence mechanisms that prevent individuals – both patients and nurses – from exploring this aspect of their lives. However, fear and ignorance will not help to eradicate or dispel myth or superstition! Allen highlights how misconception and society's perceptions can influence peoples' attitudes to this issue:

> I would probably rather tell you about my sex life than about my spiritual life. And I'm fairly sure you would be more scandalized to find a Bible at

the bottom of my brie[...]
p.52)

Research indicates that such ba[...]
external sources (Waugh 1992; M[...]
the patient or nurse themselves; an [...]
(organisational or managerial) in wh[...]
Probably by far the biggest barrier is the [...]
applies to the religious. Allen's quotation[...]
that there is still a reluctance within society [...]
spiritual matters because, for some people[...]
included), spirituality is still synonymous wit[...]
barriers the nursing profession has shown, throug[...]
that spirituality applies to all people, irrespective of [...]
atheists and agnostics included (Burnard 1988). Thro[...]
awareness raising, nurses are becoming more informed [...]
that may prevent the delivery of spiritual care.

Issues of role

A further potential barrier to spiritual care delivery by nurses relat[...]
question of whether they feel it is their role to be involved in this as[...]
care. Soeken and Carson highlight this problem:

> Meeting the spiritual needs of patients can be uncomfortable for the nurs[...]
> Several reasons for such discomforts include embarrassment, the belief
> that it is not the nurse's role, lack of training, and lack of own spiritual
> resources. (1987, p.610)

It is recognised that the provision of spiritual care can be costly both
emotionally and spiritually to the nurse (Harrison and Burnard 1993;
McSherry 2000). Yet with reference to the blurring of role, the
contemporary research referred to throughout this piece indicates that
nurses are fully aware of the boundaries that exist between themselves and
other health care professionals. They are also, it seems, aware of their own
limitations when dealing with this aspect of care. Nurses can distinguish
between a spiritual need that has its origins within a religious framework
and those that are more existential in nature. This ability to differentiate
indicates that they are acutely aware of the need for good inter-disciplinary
collaboration when dealing with this aspect of care.

two fund-
a cardiac
·aken in
rgeon,
's not
the
ife

SPIRITUAL CRISIS? CALL A NURSE / 113

(case than a copy of the Kama Sutra. (Allen 1991,
rriers can be related to both internal and
Sherry 1997). An internal source may be
external one could be the environment
ch spiritual care is being provided.
isconception that spirituality only
reinforces this point, indicating
(health care professionals
o talk freely and openly about
religion. Despite these
h dialogue and debate,
religious affiliation —
ugh education and
about the barriers

es to the
ect of

-poly
nat nurses

atients this will necessitate
g to enable patients to meet their
of the need to enlist the services of the
religious leader to meet religious needs where
they may enlist the help of another agency, with the
sent, to help deal with a spiritual need concerning bereavement
ss. A nurse may act as an advocate or facilitator to aid the patient in meeting a specific spiritual need. There can be no room for scepticism and doubt in assisting a nurse to help a patient meet their spiritual need. Collaboration by all health care professionals is required to ensure the patient achieves resolution.

Scepticism

While there is a growing realisation of the importance of spirituality to the health and well-being of patients, there remains a great deal of scepticism within medicine. Perhaps this arises because the area of spirituality is deeply subjective, personal and beyond the realms of scientific enquiry. Nurses and other health care professionals (chaplains, occupational therapists) are taking the lead, challenging the medical and scientific fraternity to reconsider the biomedical model and asking them to recognise the importance of the spiritual dimension within the lives of all individuals. If there is to be good multi-disciplinary and inter-disciplinary communication and collaboration, the medical world needs to stop, listen and evaluate its understanding of the spiritual dimension. Medicine needs to take seriously the contemporary interest in the spiritual dimension, supporting other health professionals in their attendance to this fundamental aspect of patient care. Perhaps then there will be true collaboration and partnership in care.

Summary

It has been argued that nurses have been the pioneers in generating an awareness of the importance of the spiritual dimension to the health and well-being of patients. Nurses have been proactive in trying to establish an evidence-base for the delivery of spiritual care. The emerging research suggests that nurses are not afraid to be involved in this very personal, sensitive and complex aspect of people's lives. The nursing profession has generated a dialogue which focuses on the importance of the spiritual dimension. A counter-argument may be that nurses are tinkering in an aspect of care in which they are unsuitably unqualified – and area which should be left to chaplains. However, it has been suggested that nurses are aware of professional boundaries. Nurses do not feel that they, or any other professional body, have a monopoly on this aspect of care. Instead they are calling for greater multi-disciplinary and inter-disciplinary collaboration. Presently it seems that patients who are experiencing a spiritual crisis should call for a nurse in the first instance. Perhaps this position will change with greater professional collaboration and co-operation in investigating the spiritual dimensions of care.

In conclusion, nursing cannot work alone in this complex and mysterious area. Co-operation and commitment is required from all professions involved in the delivery of health care. Nursing has thrown down the gauntlet, challenging and leading all health care professionals into a time of new spiritual growth. It is time for all to capitalise on and further develop the pioneering work undertaken. Otherwise the title of this chapter will remain a constant reality – if a patient is experiencing a spiritual crisis they will need to call a nurse.

References

Allen, C. (1991) 'The inner light.' *Nursing Standard 5*, 20, 52–53.

Balkizas, D. and O'Hare, M. (1994) 'The helping hand of God.' *Nursing Standard 9*, 9, 46–47.

Birchenall, P. (1987) 'The spiritual dimension.' In A. Parrish *Mental Handicap: The Essentials of Nursing.* London: Macmillan.

Bradshaw, A. (1994) *Lighting the Lamp: The Spiritual Dimension of Nursing Care.* London: Scutari Press.

Bradshaw, A. (1996) 'The legacy of Nightingale.' *Nursing Times 92*, 6, 42–43.

Burnard, P. (1988) 'The spiritual needs of atheists and agnostics.' *Professional Nurse*, December, 130–132.

Carson, V. B. (1989) *Spiritual Dimensions of Nursing Practice.* Philadelphia: W. B. Saunders.

Catterall, R.A., Cobb, M., Greet, B., Sankey, J. and Griffiths, G. (1998) 'The assessment and audit of spiritual care.' *International Journal of Palliative Nursing 4*, 4, 162–168.

Cawley, N. (1997) 'An exploration of the concept of spirituality.' *International Journal of Palliative Care 3*, 1, 31–36.

Cobb, M. and Robshaw, V. (1998) *The Spiritual Challenge of Health Care.* Edinburgh: Churchill Livingstone.

Department of Health (1996) *The Patient's Charter.* London: HMSO.

Farmer, E. (1996) *Exploring the Spiritual Dimension of Care.* Lancaster: Quay Books.

Griffin, A. (1993) 'Holism in nursing: its meaning and value.' *British Journal of Nursing 2*, 6, 310–312.

Ham-Ying, S. (1993) 'Analysis of the concept of holism within the context of nursing.' *British Journal of Nursing 2*, 15, 771–775.

Harrison, J. (1993) 'Spirituality and nursing practice.' *Journal of Clinical Nursing 2*, 211–217.

Harrison, J. and Burnard, P. (1993) *Spirituality and Nursing Practice.* Aldershot: Avebury.

Johnston Taylor, E., Highfield, M. and Amenta, M. (1994) 'Attitudes and beliefs regarding spiritual care.' *Cancer Nursing 17*, 6, 479–487.

Kenny, G. (1999) 'Assessing children's spirituality.' *British Journal of Nursing 8*, 1, 28–32.

Kratz, C. R. (1979) *The Nursing Process.* London: Bailliere Tindall.

Males, J. and Boswell C. (1990) 'Spiritual needs of people with a mental handicap.' *Nursing Standard 4*, 48, 35–37.

McSherry, W. (1997) 'A Descriptive Survey of Nurses' Perceptions of Spirituality and Spiritual Care.' Unpublished Master of Philosophy Thesis. University of Hull, England.

McSherry, W. (2000) *Making Sense of Spirituality in Nursing Practice: An Interactive Approach.* Edinburgh: Churchill Livingstone.

Mickley, J. R., Carson, V. and Soeken, K. L. (1995) 'Religion and adult mental health: state of the science in nursing.' *Issues in Mental Health Nursing 16*, 345–360.

Murray, R. B. and Zentner, J. B. (1989) *Nursing Concepts for Health Promotion.* London: Prentice Hall.

Narayanasamy, A. (1991) *Spiritual care: a practical guide for nurses.* Lancaster: Quay Publishing.

Narayanasamy, A. (1993) 'Nurses' awareness and educational preparation in meeting their patients' spiritual needs.' *Nurse Education Today 13,* 3, 196–201.

Narayanasamy, A. (1996) 'Spiritual care of chronically ill patients.' *British Journal of Nursing 5,* 7, 411–416.

Narayanasamy, A. (1999) 'Learning spiritual dimensions of care from a historical perspective.' *Nurse Education Today 19,* 386–395.

Oldnall, A. S. (1995) 'On the absence of spirituality in nursing theories and models.' *Journal of Advanced Nursing 21,* 417–418.

Ross, L. (1995) 'The spiritual dimension: its importance to patients' health, well-being and quality of life and its implications for nursing practice.' *International Journal of Nursing Studies 32,* 5, 457–468.

Ross, L. (1996) 'Teaching spiritual care to nurses.' *Nurse Education Today 16,* 38–43.

Ross, L. (1997) *Nurses' Perceptions of Spiritual Care.* Aldershot: Avebury.

Simsen, B. (1985) 'Spiritual needs and resources in illness and hospitalisation.' Unpublished M.Sc Thesis of the University of Manchester, England.

Soeken, K. L. and Carson, V. J. (1987) 'Responding to the spiritual needs of the chronically ill.' *Nursing Clinics of North America 22,* 3, 603–611.

Stoll, R. (1979) 'Guidelines for spiritual assessment.' *American Journal of Nursing 79,* 1574–1577.

Stoter, D. (1995) *Spiritual Aspects of Health Care.* London: Mosby.

Swaffield, L. (1988) 'Religious roots.' *Nursing Times 84,* 28–30.

Waugh, L. A. (1992) 'Spiritual aspects of nursing: a descriptive study of nurses' perceptions.' Unpublished PhD Thesis of Queen Margaret College, Edinburgh, Scotland.

CHAPTER 9

Towards Competence
A Narrative and Framework for Spiritual Care Givers

Martin Kerry

The national context

In broad terms, *competencies* are 'the skills, knowledge, experience, attributes and behaviours that an individual needs to perform a job effectively' (Strebler, Thompson and Heron 1997, p.12). A wide range of organisations have used them for human resource purposes including appraisal, selection, training and development and determining pay levels. Competencies differ from appraisal mechanisms such as individual performance review in their focus on inputs as well as outputs. They are concerned with how employees

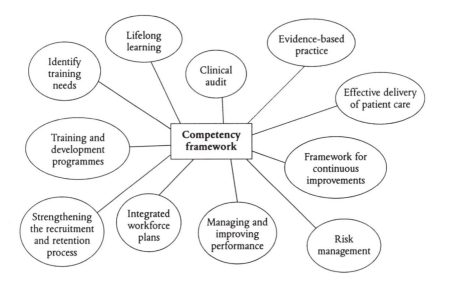

Figure 9.1 Links between a competency framework and clinical governance

go about their job – their behaviour in fulfilling a particular role – as well as reviewing the objectives towards which they work.

Clinical governance has been central to the Labour government's drive to define, develop and deliver excellence in clinical care (Department of Health 1998). It is a framework for improved practice and accountability as well as increasing professionalism. A competency approach can be seen as a key mechanism for delivering clinical governance (see Figure 9.1). It links to personnel issues such as strengthening recruitment and retention. It relates directly to the training and development processes required for Investors in People accreditation. It offers a structure for continuous improvement supporting clinical audit and risk management.

Whilst competencies were initially used in the NHS as a way of assessing and developing managers, they have more recently been embraced by a wide range of clinical staff as a way of delivering the clinical governance agenda.

Health care chaplaincy essayed its own description of competencies at a relatively early date. The *Healthcare Chaplaincy Standards* (NHSTD 1993) offers 'a definition of competent performance in the workplace'. 'Each of the components of a work role is described in terms of the outcomes that should be achieved, and the range of situations in which a competent practitioner would be expected to perform.' I personally have quarried the *Standards* in order to formulate job descriptions, to identify training and development needs, and as a source of language for communicating with managers about the purpose and aspirations of chaplaincy. However, the *Standards* has not won the hearts and minds of chaplains in general, nor has it been integrated into the practice of very many chaplaincy departments. This may derive from the language and structure of the material which could be perceived as culturally alien to chaplaincy. There are over 30 pages listing 'performance criteria' of elements of competence. At first sight these say little about the qualities of being and attitude that chaplains have traditionally regarded as central to their role.

This chapter presents an account of one attempt to develop health care chaplaincy/spiritual care standards for a local context. The context is a large district general hospital: Nottingham City Hospital NHS Trust. The account aims to be accessible enough to be of practical use on the ground, as well as reflecting contemporary national interest in competency frameworks as a key contribution to clinical governance.

Local development

In the first instance it is necessary to describe the drivers, principles and process underlying the development of the competency framework for chaplaincy at Nottingham City Hospital.

Drivers

The drivers for any change need to be of sufficient weight to overcome the resistance that almost invariably attends change. There were several drivers for developing the framework. The first of these was recruitment and retention issues in chaplaincy. Three of the four full-time chaplains were employed at 'assistant grade' (a pay scale of just three increments) leaving the postholder significantly worse off financially than, say, a team vicar. Understandably, staff were inclined to look for a move after three or four years, and attracting high calibre new staff proved difficult.

The second driver was the human resources agenda to introduce local pay. This was to be based on competency progression rather than automatic incremental advancement. In other words, a postholder would need to demonstrate development in his or her job role in order to progress to the next level of the pay scale. This provided a means of extending the assistant chaplain's pay spine from its current nationally determined NHS level to a point almost equivalent to the bottom of the 'whole-time' (more senior) scale. In effect, a chaplain who was happy to remain in the job for all other reasons would now not need to leave in order to advance their pay. A prerequisite for competency progression was the development of a competency framework. This caught the tide of a gathering body of work on competencies across the Trust. Competency schemes were being introduced in theatres, rehabilitation and some areas of nursing; an ambitious project had recently begun to introduce a single competency framework for Professions Allied to Medicine (PAMS); and a day conference on competencies was organised for all Trust managers.

The main resistances to change derived from the increased funding required to extend pay spines, and from a diffidence amongst chaplains to assessment and evaluation of their performance. The drivers ensured both the political will at Trust level, and an incentive at the level of the individual chaplain and chaplaincy department, to overcome these blocks to implementation.

Principles

Two key principles underpinned the way in which the competency framework was developed. Chaplaincy and spiritual care are an integral part of the hospital's endeavour to heal, care and rehabilitate. A necessary corollary of this is that chaplaincy is willing to engage with the organisational processes of the hospital as fully as any other hospital

---

1. **Research**
    - competency frameworks already developed at NCH by other professionals
    - Health care Chaplaincy Standards (NHSTD 1993)
    - background articles on competencies
    - other written resources e.g. Chaplaincy Department Service Profile, job descriptions
    - work at national level via Hospital Chaplaincies Council

2. **Consult**
    - ongoing dialogue between Personnel Adviser and Senior Chaplain who managed the whole process
    - with staff at NCH who were working with competencies
    - with Professional Development Officer at the Hospital Chaplaincies Council
    - with the chaplaincy team: involved at all stages

3. **Implement**
    - framework produced in draft form – consultation reiterated
    - final version of framework
    - baseline assessment (May/June 2000) – strengths affirmed – key areas for growth identified
    - Professional Development Plans produced for each chaplain – revisited at monthly reviews
    - assessment process for next year agreed.

4. **Evaluate**
    - with all involved in implementation
    - with chaplaincy colleagues in Trent Region e.g. study day with presentation and discussion
    - will lead to further development and refinement.

Figure 9.2 Process of developing the competency framework

department, and that chaplains are subject to the same degree of rigour in working through the implications of clinical governance as other professionals. Consistency with other professional groups was therefore one guiding principle.

In any process of change the involvement of those most affected (in the formulation of goals and methods) is desirable both philosophically and pragmatically. Such an approach leads to *empowerment*, encouraging the taking of responsibility; *ownership*, harnessing everyone's creative contribution; and the *removal of suspicion/fear*, thus dissolving resistance to change. This sort of involvement is possible at local level in a way that a national endeavour such as *Healthcare Chaplaincy Standards* cannot replicate, making it the key difference between the two. The involvement of the chaplaincy team was therefore a second basic principle.

Process

The process of developing the framework in Nottingham is summarised in Figure 9.2. The main phases in the process were: Research, Consult, Implement and Evaluate.

A vital aspect of the process has been working through the two above-mentioned principles. For example, the first principle – the desire for consistency with other professionals – informed the structuring of the framework. The framework consists of three major categories of competency: knowledge, behaviour and skills. These reflect the approach of a local PAMS project as well as the emerging norm in other disciplines.

The framework operates at three *levels* of competency. Locally, nursing had adapted the work of Benner (1984) to develop the following three-stage model.

				Level 3
		Level 2	$\rightarrow$	Expert Practitioner
	$\rightarrow$	Proficient Practitioner		Proficient Practitioner
Level 1		Competent Practitioner		
Advanced Beginner		Advanced Beginner		
Novice				

(Source: Elaine Wilson)

These three levels were applied to chaplaincy as follows:

Level 1: Part-time chaplains and newly appointed whole-time assistant chaplains

Level 2: Whole-time assistants and whole-time chaplains in smaller Trusts

Level 3: Whole-time chaplains managing teams or with extended responsibility

With regard to the second principle, involvement, the chaplaincy team participated in debating, accepting and moulding the structure of the framework and, crucially, in developing its content. The central question: 'What does a good one look like?' was applied throughout. Chaplains know what a good chaplain is, just as nurses know what a good nurse is.

For each area of competence the team was asked to generate examples with positive and negative indicators so that performance could be demonstrated and evaluated. A simple instance can be seen in the 'worship' area of competence. This lists five skills: planning, liturgical, analytical, pastoral and facilitative. The entry for 'planning' reads:

Example	*Positive indicator*	*Negative indicator*
Organises personnel, environment and materials for effective worship.	e.g. order of service produced on time.	e.g. organists not informed of music.

Introducing the framework

Overview

The chaplaincy competency framework has three *categories* (knowledge, behaviour, skills) operating at three *levels* of practitioner. Figure 9.3 gives an overview of the framework with the headline areas of competence.

The *knowledge* category actually contains 12–15 areas of competence for each of Levels 1–3. It also includes a 'basic' level for volunteer chaplaincy workers and theological students.

Category	Level indicator	Areas of competence
1. Knowledge	Basic (voluntary pastoral visitors, theological students)	NHS background, people who work in hospital, hospitalisation etc.
	Level 1 (sessional chaplains, new assistant chaplains)	Departmental processes, professional roles, bereavement theory etc.
	Level 2 (experienced chaplains)	Hospital-wide structures and processes, non-Christian faiths, ethical theory etc.
	Level 3 (team leaders, expert practitioners)	National processes, external agencies, management theory etc.
2. Behaviour	Equally applicable to all levels, but chaplains are expected to demonstrate a continuous process of development in each area	Reflective, Spiritual, Accepting, Creative, Self-aware, Other-aware, Available, Reliable, Versatile, Communicative
3. Skills	Clinical	Pastoral, Worship, Bereavement
	Resourcing	Theological/Ethical, Supervision, Training and Development
	Generic	Personal, Departmental, Organisational, External

Figure 9.3 Overview of competency framework

The *behaviour* category contains ten areas. Each describes the attitudes, personal qualities and 'ways of being' which impact upon the way chaplaincy is carried out. They reflect the belief that the whole person of the chaplain mediates effective care, and are an attempt to make explicit the attributes which are for the most part implicit in *Healthcare Chaplaincy Standards*.

The *skills* category requires further explanation in terms of three sub-categories. The skills required in the 'clinical' sub-category are chaplaincy-specific. They relate to the core work of pastoral care, worship, bereavement and loss. The skills in the 'generic' sub-category include consultation, profiling and strategy and are not limited to chaplaincy but are employed in a wide range of jobs. They are arranged like concentric circles in terms of broadening areas of work (personal, departmental, organisational, external). The outward movement reflects the changing arenas of the work of chaplains as they move into leadership and management. The skills required in the 'resourcing' sub-category combine elements of both of the other two. Typically the skills are generic but are applied with a chaplaincy-specific knowledge and awareness. Chaplains operating at Levels 1–3 need differing degrees of proficiency and have distinctive emphases in their focus of work across these sub-categories (see Figure 9.4). For example, a Level 3 chaplain with more managerial scope will require greater proficiency in skills such as profiling or strategic vision.

	Proficiency required			Focus of work
	Clinical skills	Resourcing skills	Generic skills	
Level 1	high	low	low	spends most time in clinical activities
Level 2	high	mid	mid	spends an increasing amount of time in 'resourcing' and 'generic' activities
Level 3	high	high	high	Spends a little time in clinical, some time in resourcing, and much time in generic activities

Figure 9.4 Relationship between level of practitioner and skills needed

As has already been indicated, each area of competence is expanded, sometimes using examples for clarification and always listing positive and negative indicators so that there is a concrete way in which performance can be evaluated. Each of the headings in the overview therefore generates a significant body of text. The examples and indicators are not intended to be exhaustive – individuals may have different ways of demonstrating a particular competency – but they are sufficiently detailed and specific to give a clear idea of what is expected.

Using the framework

The framework is intended to follow an annual cycle. Following a first-year baseline assessment exercise, an annual assessment is completed each March. Chaplains who can demonstrate progression to an agreed degree of competence subsequently advance by one pay point.

The process of assessment works in the following way. The chaplain to be assessed works through the entire framework, annotating the text with comments of assessment. The chaplain then gives a copy to his or her line manager (e.g. the senior chaplain for assistant chaplains) who also works through the framework. This is followed by a two-hour interview between the chaplain and the line manager. The manager focuses on strengths to be affirmed, developmental needs, and areas where there is a discrepancy between the assessment made by the manager and that of the chaplain. The discrepancies generate a discussion in which issues can be explored. At the end of the interview, areas for development are mutually agreed. These comprise a maximum of two areas from each of the three categories of the framework. The chaplain is then asked to develop these into a Personal Development Plan with SMART (Specific, Measurable, Achievable, Relevant, Time-limited) objectives. Achievement of the plan becomes the focus of next year's assessment, although competencies across the whole framework will be reviewed and progress in other areas can be acknowledged. The chaplain is responsible for compiling a portfolio of evidence to demonstrate proficiency (e.g. courses attended, evaluation forms from training sessions given, logs of committees or working groups with samples of any written contributions).

The process for achieving the plan is intended to be dynamic and flexible. For example, at Nottingham City Hospital all chaplains have individual monthly supervision meetings with their manager, where progress with the competencies can be reviewed and emerging issues can be integrated into the existing plan, renegotiating goals where necessary.

Two examples from practice

Training and development is an area of competence within the 'resourcing skills' sub-category (see Figure 9.5).

TRAINING AND DEVELOPMENT

Overall Aim:	to initiate and contribute to training and development in chaplaincy-related issues
Range:	Volunteers, students, hospital staff bereavement, spiritual needs, religions...

Skill	Example	Positive indicator	Negative indicator
Analytical	Identifies training needs and training opportunities, especially in own area of responsibility	Is proactive in seeking opportunities to offer T&D	Is passive in respect of T&D
Planning and composition	Evolves, adapts and develops a portfolio of topics	Has a developing portfolio	Lack of portfolio or static portfolio
Teaching skills	Can deliver material imaginatively and in a manner tailored to clients	Positive evluation of clients	Negative evaluation of clients

Figure 9.5 Entry for Training and Development area of competence

The skills required are generic, but chaplaincy-specific knowledge and experience are needed for the context in which they are applied. One chaplain identified this area as 'the one I am weakest in'. This did not conflict with expectations since he had only been a chaplain for 15 months. The competency framework identifies this as the transition time from Level 1 to Level 2, the 'Advanced Beginner', and would accordingly expect him only to be beginning to develop Resourcing and Generic skills, and to start spending an increasing amount of time in these activities (see Figure 9.4).

Further discussion elicited subtle distinctions between the three subsets of skills. On enquiry, he had responded to occasional requests for training input on bereavement, the role of the chaplaincy and so on, and he already had an embryonic portfolio of topics 'planning and composition'. The element yet to happen was the 'analytical' identification of where he could offer training inputs within his areas of responsibility in the hospital. He also felt he lacked confidence in his 'teaching skills', which impeded his progress in the outworking of the other two skills.

The chaplain and his manager explored these issues, and ways of responding to them emerged. 'Training and development' was identified as an area for growth along with three or four areas from other sections of the competency framework. The chaplain was asked to produce a draft Personal Development Plan for the year ahead, which was discussed and refined at a subsequent meeting. To address the training and development competency, a set of actions was agreed. These included attending training on presentation skills to improve teaching confidence; ensuring feedback and evaluation are received on any teaching and training activities and recording these for discussion. In addition, appropriate opportunities for hands-on experience of training in his areas of work are to be identified, with the aim of both developing the chaplain's skills and resourcing staff. The chaplain will look to extend gradually the range of topics he can offer, and progress will be reviewed as part of the monthly supervision sessions held regularly with the line manager. There is a clear emphasis here on the inputs required to do the job effectively, although performance (outputs) will be evaluated at the next annual assessment.

The process of reviewing competencies also alerted the chaplaincy manager to make a shift in his expectations of the chaplain from 'Novice' to 'Advanced Beginner', so that, for example, when requests to provide training come into the department, the manager now considers this chaplain more actively.

The second example is taken from the 'behaviour' area of competence. The entry for 'available' reads:

Example	Positive indicator	Negative indicator
Maintains a presence on wards. Responds to referrals within appropriate time. Welcomes droppers-in	Offers a physical and emotional availability to colleagues and clients.	Staff and patients unaware of chaplaincy. Chaplain perceived as having a 'remote' persona.

The chaplain's own annotations indicated an awareness that she was not visiting some of her wards as much as was required. Interestingly this point complemented issues raised elsewhere in the competency framework – for example, a gap in training and development initiatives – demonstrating the value of the framework in building up an 'identikit' picture of the chaplain in her job. This led to discussion around the reasons for not visiting: partly the busyness of some weeks, partly a lack of focus by the chaplain which in its turn derived from the fact that she had never really felt established on these wards.

The chaplain identified two wards on which to focus initially. She would arrange interviews with the ward managers in order to discuss profiling chaplaincy (perhaps via ward meetings), training and development needs and ward expectations of the chaplaincy service. She would also keep a log of pastoral visits made to these wards. The success criteria would be whether after six months the chaplain was known to staff, and whether referrals increased from these wards.

These decisions were documented in the chaplain's Personal Development Plan. At the next monthly supervision session she was able to report early success – one of the ward managers had referred a member of staff for counselling.

Taking the framework forward

Evaluation

The final element in the process of developing the competency framework is evaluation (see Figure 9.2 above). Once again, it was vital to take seriously the experience of those involved. The reflections of the chaplains who have actually used the framework have obviously been important. We have learned through doing and then reflecting on what we have done. All those who had been consulted initially were asked to evaluate the framework in its final form. In addition, a wider consultation was begun amongst chaplains across the NHS region of Trent through presentations and various forums.

Findings so far

Although the *structure* of the framework appears extremely robust and viable, it is clear that further refinement of the *content* is needed. In particular, the positive and negative indicators do not always work constructively. On occasion, they merely present opposites without developing the sense of the competency. For example, the theological/ethical area of competence in the skills category requires *inter alia* 'presentation skills'. At present the positive indicator reads, 'effectiveness of presentation' and the negative, 'ineffectiveness of presentation'

A second issue concerns the assessment of the senior chaplain. The line manager to this post is the Director of Nursing, who feels competent to assess generic competencies, but not chaplaincy-specific ones. The way forward here may be either to construct the evidence for fulfilment of the competency in a way which can be grasped by the Director; or to invite a peer chaplain to carry out the assessment of clinical areas. The problem is not dissimilar to that faced by other professions.

Several benefits are emerging. First, the competency framework offers a means of articulating *shared expectations* around performance. The chaplains who took part were surprised at how liberating this proved. Rather than experiencing these expectations as a threat, they found it immensely useful to have a yardstick and picture of what it meant to be a good chaplain. Frequently, this allowed strengths to be appreciated much more explicitly than would have been the case without a framework. It also enabled areas for development to be explored in a non-threatening, non-accusatory manner.

The framework provides a text in a mutually agreed language (and hence more useful than the *Healthcare Chaplaincy Standards*) which can nonetheless be interpreted flexibly for individual application. Since the framework and the individual personal development plans generated from it have been formed collaboratively, there is effectively a *contract* for delivering quality and professionalism.

It is also increasingly clear that the competency framework provides a tool for ensuring continuity in professional development. Previously, objectives from appraisals were reviewed annually and new goals were set for the following year. However, there was no year-on-year sense of direction other than those provided by individual or departmental objectives. Now development is encouraged in the context of an overarching framework that consistently presents a picture of what a good professional chaplain looks like.

Finally, there is a growing confidence that the framework, in conjunction with local pay, will deliver on the original driver of strengthening retention and recruitment. There is less pressure to seek a move on grounds of pay alone. When recruitment is necessary, the framework will be invaluable in writing job descriptions and in providing a pay incentive for applicants.

Hopes for the future

I hope that this narrative may inspire others to develop their own competency frameworks. It will not be possible simply to apply the Nottingham City Hospital version, since an integral part of development comprises the inductive process of its formulation. Some work will need to be done from 'inside-out'.

One of the criticisms which has been levelled at the competency approach generally is that by basing definitions of competence on current and past practice, innovation is stifled and future possibilities are constricted, looking to do no more than clone successors (IDS 1997). By taking an inductive approach and giving the current chaplaincy team a pivotal role in defining the content of the framework, we have run this risk. I would hope to counter it with wider continuing dialogue. This will be dialogue with national standards. In fact the local framework we produced was always aware of the *Healthcare Chaplaincy Standards* and the skills section, in particular, draws from them. They offer an important external (perhaps more objective) perspective. Future versions of the standards will inform the Nottingham City Hospital framework – and I hope vice versa.

It will also be further dialogue with chaplaincy users. 'What do you think a good one looks like?', will add an important dimension and ensure that the framework is vital and relevant.

And it will be dialogue with other health care professionals. I hope the chaplaincy framework provides a sufficiently common language and structure to contribute constructively to the task of interdisciplinary conversation. This is very important in an NHS where the goal of collaboration for patient benefit is still stifled by professional insularity. Competency frameworks from across disciplines could promote mutual understanding of roles and aspirations.

It seems likely that the chaplaincy competency framework will make a significant contribution to clinical governance; improving the performance of chaplains so that care for patients, relatives and staff benefits in a practical way as well as enhancing the professionalism of chaplaincy so that spiritual care may take its place as an integral part of the healing endeavour in the modern NHS.

Acknowledgements

The author wishes to thank the following for permission to use their unpublished material in this chapter:

Elaine Wilson, Senior Nurse Manager Cancer Services Division, Nottingham City Hospital, for Figure 9.1 and the '3 levels of competency' diagram.

Malcolm Masterman, formerly Professional Development Officer at the Hospital Chaplaincies Council, for material from a Training Standards Working Group on which the 'knowledge' category of the competency framework is based.

References

Benner, P. (1984) *From Novice to Expert: Excellence and Power in Clinical Nursing Practice.* San Francisco: Addison-Wesley Publishing Co.

Department of Health (1998) *A First Class Service – Quality in the New NHS.* London: Department of Health.

Incomes Data Services (1997) *Developing Competency Frameworks, Incomes Data Services, Study 639.* London: Incomes Data Services Ltd.

NHS Training Directorate (1993) *Healthcare Chaplaincy Standards.* Bristol: NHS Training Directorate.

Strebler, M. Thompson, M. and Heron, P. (1997) *Skills, Competencies and Gender: Issues for Pay and Training.* Report 333. Brighton: Institute for Employment Studies.

PART THREE
Cultural Contexts

CHAPTER 10

Sociological Perspectives on the Pastoral Care of Minority Faiths in Hospital[1]

Sophie Gilliat-Ray

A West African woman who spoke no English refused to eat in hospital. Every time she was offered food she would shake her head and chant 'ramadan-ramadan-ramadan'. The staff didn't understand that she was observing the Muslim fast of Ramadan and could therefore only eat during the hours of darkness. They thought she was mad. (Interview with a nursery nurse, cited in Schott and Henley 1996, p.12)

When I went into hospital I only got vegetarian food. After a few days I realised other people were getting more interesting meals. When I asked I discovered that it was because I had given my religion as Muslim. I was brought up a Muslim but I'm not at all religious. I thought you had to give an answer and I didn't know what else to say. (Interview with an Iranian woman, cited in Schott and Henley 1996, p.13)

Ignorance and stereotyped assumptions on the part of nursing staff are just some of the barriers hindering more inclusive and appropriate care for religious minority groups in hospitals. Lack of awareness about religious and cultural diversity held by many hospital staff reflects the fact that the quality of care given to patients from minority faith traditions is often shaped by a complex interplay of sociological and contextual factors. This chapter will explore some of the issues that affect the care of religious minorities in hospital by examining issues of power and empowerment, authority, equality and representation. I shall also be considering how the wider social context *outside* hospitals to some extent affects the care they receive *within* health care institutions. Likewise, the internal dynamics and politics of hospitals must be considered in terms of their influence upon the way patients from minority traditions are regarded, both individually and collectively.

To begin the discussion we need to step back one decade to the launch of *The Patient's Charter* in 1991. This document marked the first significant political recognition of religious diversity in health care. As part of a wider government initiative to improve the quality of services that citizens received from the state, *The Patient's Charter* established a number of criteria by which this might be assessed in the field of health care. The first of nine National Charter Standards specified the right of patients to 'respect for privacy, dignity, and religious and cultural beliefs'. For the first time, a concern for the spiritual and religious welfare of patients was incumbent on all NHS staff, not just chaplains, and no distinction was made between Christian and non-Christian patients. The onus was placed on managers to either employ qualified staff to meet the spiritual needs of patients and staff; to contract with relevant organisations for the provision of sessional spiritual care; or to facilitate voluntary visits by religious leaders to patients from their tradition. Managers could take account of the make-up of the local religious community in deciding which of these three options represented the most appropriate action, introducing a new degree of flexibility into arrangements for spiritual and religious care. Much of this chapter will try to answer the question as to how far the ideals embodied in *The Patient's Charter* have translated into an equitable reality for members of minority traditions.

Pastoral care for religious minorities: factors external to the hospital

In the absence of reliable data, the composition of Britain's major faith traditions is estimated in *Religions in the UK: a Multi-Faith Directory* (Weller 1997, p.29) as follows:[2] Bahai's – 6000; Buddhists – 30,000–130,000; Christians – 40,000,000; Hindus – 400,000–500,000; Jains – 25,000–30,000; Jews – 300,000; Muslims – 1,000,000–1,500,000; Sikhs – 350,000–500,000, Zoroastrians – 5000–10,000. These populations are not monolithic entities; all the major faith traditions in Britain are characterised by an internal diversity of language, ethnicity, race, gender, age, class, and membership of different philosophical schools of thought. Additionally, their geographic distribution around the country is uneven, with the highest concentrations of religious diversity in large industrial towns and cities.[3] Many of the adherents of minority faith communities are also members of ethnic or racial minority groups. This being the case, they may be confronted by a range of difficulties in their interaction with health care institutions that may be specific to their membership of linguistic or racial minority groups, rather than their membership of a religious community. Examples include disadvantage or discrimination when it comes to access to health information in community languages; identifying, recording and using names correctly; providing suitable menus, and so on. This chapter is specifically concerned with those aspects of care that relate to membership of a religious minority group.

The provision of pastoral care to Christian patients, nominal or otherwise, is most likely to come from whole- or part-time Christian chaplains or clergy employed by the hospital or trust. It is now increasingly recognised that minority faith traditions do not have a formal tradition of 'chaplaincy', nor do they have personnel who function as an approximate equivalent to a chaplain (Schott and Henley 1996; Gilliat-Ray 2000). Though Jewish rabbis in Britain have gradually incorporated a pastoral dimension to their role, it is only in the past few years that numerically larger minority traditions, such as Islam, have been drawn into chaplaincy or pastoral work on a significant scale. Reflecting the traditions of the countries from which Britain's Buddhist, Hindu, Muslim, Sikh and other faiths have originated, spiritual support has largely come from family members, not from full-time religious professionals. However, a combination of factors is changing this situation.

First, the extended family system upon which most emotional and spiritual support has depended in minority faith communities is coming under a number of pressures. The extended family is less able to provide either practical or pastoral care support as its traditional structure fragments under the influence of social and geographic mobility and change (Berthoud and Beishon 1997).

Second, since other faith traditions do not traditionally have personnel who function as chaplains, it is becoming clear that if they are to engage with public institutions in Britain that *do* employ chaplains, it is necessary to promote some religious professionals or community leaders into the proximal role of 'chaplain'. This has become such a feature of the development of modern chaplaincy that I shall refer to it by the term 'approximation'.[4] The process of approximation refers to changing religious roles within a tradition engendered by contact with a dominant religious tradition. Professional pastoral roles that already exist in the 'host' context have a determining influence on how other faiths *without* such roles engage in public institutions. The 'traditional' role adapts to the 'host' role. Thus, many religious professionals or community leaders from minority faith groups are gradually extending the remit of their work under the combined pressure of hospital expectations, the lack of other alternative personnel, and the fragmentation of extended family support networks.

Despite nationwide evidence for incremental 'approximation', given the uneven geographical distribution of faith communities in Britain, the availability of local religious or community leaders who can provide 'spiritual care' for members of religious minority groups will depend, at least partially, on geography. No matter how well-intentioned hospital managers or chaplains might be to 'facilitate' professional pastoral care, members of minority traditions who are hospitalised away from larger concentrations of fellow-believers and/or places of worship, are unlikely to have their needs met by a religious professional or community leader from their own tradition. During the 'Church of England and Other Faiths Project', at least one of the frustrations expressed by hospital chaplains when it came to facilitating pastoral care for patients from minority traditions was 'getting hold of other faith representatives to come into the hospital' and 'accessing appropriate 'leaders' from ethnic communities to serve as part of the chaplaincy team'. At least some of the reason for their frustration was due to the simple fact of the geographical location of the hospital relative to sizeable local faith communities.

Issues of gender are also significant in terms of the availability and/or suitability of religious or community personnel to visit hospital patients from their tradition. The vast majority of faith community leaders are male. Social and religious norms in some traditions prohibit unrelated men and women meeting alone, and some priests or imams are reluctant to engage in 'pastoral care' for female patients. This would prohibit female patients from comfortably sharing any private emotional or spiritual concerns with a religious professional from their community. In such instances, they may feel infinitely more comfortable confiding in a female Christian chaplain, but patient choice is one of the underpinning principles of *The Patient's Charter*.

Recognition of gender issues is now starting to shape developments in modern chaplaincy. In the Summer of 2000, Birmingham Women's Health Care NHS Trust advertised for the appointment of a 'Muslim Chaplain (Female)'.[5] From this example, not only is the process of approximation evident – in the creation of a new kind of Muslim religious professional role – but the particular needs of women from the Islamic tradition have been recognised. A similar role for a 'Muslim Chaplain (Male)' was advertised by

University Hospital Birmingham NHS Trust a few months later. It remains to be seen whether the needs of other women, perhaps from the various Indian religious traditions, will be met by the creation of similar posts. Achieving equity between minority traditions might become a challenge for the Trust.

Leaving aside the question of geography and gender, hospital managers and chaplains keen to build a multi-faith chaplaincy 'team' have sometimes failed to recognise a number of other issues, internal to faith communities, which affects the degree to which they are willing or able to participate in pastoral care. For example, some religious leaders may be poorly remunerated for their services to their own communities or places of worship, reflecting the level of poverty within the ethnic groups that support them (Berthoud 1997; Runnymede Trust 2000). If their services to the hospital are expected to be voluntary – as they often are; if the system for claiming expenses is complicated or not readily understandable (volunteers may have a limited facility in English); if there are already many pressures upon their time; and if pastoral care for individuals is seen as relatively unimportant when their wider community is facing larger crises or issues, the result does not need explanation.

In the face of these apparent challenges, the efforts of Birmingham NHS Trust and one or two other Trusts around the country, to employ and properly remunerate part- or whole-time chaplaincy posts for members of other faiths, is a welcome development. The more complex question of whether these faith communities and/or post-holders might feel that Christian patterns of pastoral care (not to mention the terminology of 'chaplaincy') are being imposed upon them, or whether they regard the process and consequences of approximation as a natural part of adaptation to a society whose traditions are underpinned by Christianity, is another matter.

Spiritual care for religious minorities: factors internal to the hospital

The previous paragraphs have already raised the issue of initiatives that hospitals might consider when it comes to enabling patients to derive spiritual care via religious professionals from their own tradition. However, recognition of the needs of religious minority groups and the quality of care they receive in hospital is subject to a wide range of other factors and influences *internal* to the life of the hospital.

As noted at the beginning of this chapter, *The Patient's Charter* was significant for placing responsibility for 'respect for religious and cultural beliefs' on all NHS staff, not just chaplains or religious professionals. Whilst nurses remain the personnel with whom patients are likely to have the greatest contact whilst in hospital, the training they receive as part of their preparation for working in a multi-faith health care environment is an important consideration. Unfortunately, hospitals remain sites where examples of cultural racism on the part of individuals and institutional discrimination more generally are evident. The recent Runnymede Trust report *The Future of Multi-Ethnic Britain* (2000) found that for members of Asian and black communities, 'there is much insensitivity in the NHS to their distinctive experiences, situations and requirements' (p.177). Documentation received for the Runnymede Trust report *Islamophobia* in 1997 gives a particularly graphic illustration of what this might entail.

> When I was in hospital recently one of the Muslim patients prayed five times a day. She either drew the curtains round her bed or went into the TV room if it was empty. The other patients laughed at her and made rude comments, and *the nurses did nothing to try and stop them*. Of course she was very hurt and upset. (Runnymede Trust 1997, p.36, emphasis added)

Of all the different reactions and responses we might have to this example, one question that comes to mind is 'How, if at all, were these nurses trained to work in a multi-faith environment, and by whom?'. At present, the kind of education about other faiths that nurses receive during their training appears to be limited to occasional lectures on death, dying and bereavement, and, in some cases, a lecture, perhaps lasting a few hours (often delivered by the hospital chaplain), about the main customs and beliefs of different faiths.[6] However, it is the written resources generated by and for the nursing profession about the religious and spiritual care of patients that helps to explain why, in some cases, the care of religious minority groups suffers because of inaccurate information and stereotyped assumptions.

Let me explain what I mean. Tucked away in the text or the appendices of a number of books on religion, spirituality and nursing there is often a 'checklist' of key beliefs and practices for the main world religions (e.g. Narayanasamy 1991; Sampson 1982). In contrast to a secularised generic 'spirituality' (see Chapter 2 by Pattison in this volume), which is assumed to be meaningful to Christians or to the general population at large, 'religion' of a committed and orthodox kind defines the so-called 'spiritual needs' of religious minority groups. To give you an example, this is what

Naranayasamy (1991) has to say about the specific religious needs of Muslims. This is taken directly out of his book; I have underlined those sections where there are difficulties.

Muslim

Birth:	May refuse internal examination. Circumcision prayer recited to baby as soon as possible.
Abortion/family planning:	Not generally disapproved of, but Muslim women think it is their duty or role in life to bear children.
Transfusion:	Generally accepted.
Diet:	Muslims eat only 'halal' meal (sic). May be vegetarian. Food regulations are strict; no pork, no alcohol. Observe Ramadan.
Death:	Opposed to post mortems. Must adhere to specific patient's religious duties. Koran (sic) recited by a relative. Family attend to duties while conforming to legal regulations. Usual for family to wash and prepare body; if not, other people wear gloves. Burial within 24 hours.
Other:	Belief that everyone is accountable to God for what he does on earth and when he dies he will be judged or punished in life hereafter. Patient will want to face 'Mecca'. A local Imam (spiritual leader) may be contacted for advice.

(Narayanasamy 1991)

Readers who know a little about Islam will immediately spot several serious misunderstandings and errors about the religious life of Muslims that could lead nurses to offer less rather than more appropriate care to Muslims.

First, the 'prayer' recited immediately after birth is the 'Call to Prayer' (the *adhan*); this prayer has no connection with circumcision whatever. Second, while family planning might be acceptable for some Muslims, abortion is only sanctioned in very particular circumstances, usually when the mental or physical health of the mother or well-being of the child is in danger. This is very different from 'not generally disapproved of'. Third, it is a serious over-generalisation to assume that all Muslim women regard their main duty or role in life to be childbearing. Some might; others might not.

Fourth, not all Muslims are strict about 'halal' food or, more particularly, halal meat. Some will accept meat that has been slaughtered by the 'People of the Book' i.e. Christians or Jews. Fifth, not all Muslims observe Ramadan, and in a textbook on nursing, surely it would have been appropriate to identify those circumstances or medical conditions that exempt Muslims from fasting (e.g. pregnancy, diabetes, liver/kidney complaints, young children, very elderly etc.). Sixth, under 'Other', the mention that Muslims will 'want to face Mecca' gives the impression that Muslims want to be permanently orientated in a south-easterly direction! The specific injunction that Muslims face Makkah (Mecca) during prayer, or for burial, is important qualifying information that was omitted.

These kinds of checklists present a very stereotyped picture of the needs of patients from different faith communities, and may lead nurses to take an over-generalised approach to the care of patients from these traditions. The dangers of this, and the possibilities for causing offence or embarrassment, are self-evident. Critiques of this approach both within and outside the nursing profession itself are few and far between, though Gerrish (1997), Lea (1994), and Walter (1997) are exceptions,[7] and works by Schott and Henley (1996; Henley and Schott 1999) represent rare examples of more useful texts for the nursing and midwifery professions. Gerrish writes:

> the underlying assumption that individuals within cultural groups share the same beliefs and values which, once identified, can be applied to other members of that culture...takes no account of the fact that diversity may exist not only between cultures but also within a culture and between generations. (1997)

The reproduction of misleading stereotypes reflects the fact that so far, minority groups do not appear to have been able to influence the discourse or dominant paradigms in nursing, or in health care planning, organisation or administration. Additionally, rates of recruitment from ethnic minorities into nursing and allied professions remain low: 'analysis of membership of the councils of the various Royal Colleges indicates an almost total absence of Asian or African surnames...medical and nursing schools are the key gatekeepers for the clinical workforce in the NHS, but the gates are not yet equitably open' (Runnymede Trust 2000, p.189). Ideally this situation will change in the future, but while stereotypes abound, it is likely to be more difficult for busy nurses, once they know a patient is a Muslim or a Hindu, to take an individualised approach to their care. In the wrong hands, these 'checklists' represent a top-down imposition of assumptions, not a negotiation of care based upon individual needs.

Some of the factors influencing pastoral care for members of different traditions are generic, affecting most minority faith groups equally. Examples include access to worship spaces free of symbols from another tradition; respectful handling of sacred texts by staff; information about religious facilities; or out-patient appointments that avoid major religious festivals. Other factors are particular to an individual faith community, such as the availability of facilities for Muslim ritual ablution before prayer. Whether generic or particular, it was clear from the research conducted as part of the 'Church of England and Other Faiths Project' that hospital and chaplaincy structures are sometimes inflexible and insensitive to the needs of patients from other faiths. Some chaplaincies and hospitals are also unaware or indifferent to the kind of measures that might significantly improve the opportunities for religious or community leaders to meet patient needs effectively.

For example, the project found that few of the faith community 'contacts' were named or mentioned in printed information about facilities available to patients belonging to traditions other than the Christian. The informality of the arrangement whereby many faith community 'contacts' are associated with chaplaincies means that they may have little or no access to patient records.[8] Although rules about confidentiality must be observed, without accurate information about the location within the hospital of patients from their tradition, their task is made more difficult. This informality can also be disempowering in other respects. For example, they may not receive adequate 'induction' about the life and norms of the hospital. They may not be invited to chaplaincy team meetings where they might contribute to decision making.[9] Few faith community leaders have a role in nurse training, and the involvement they do have tends to be one-off and brief.[10] They may not be consulted about the use of worship facilities,[11] and so on. Perhaps more significantly, these examples signify a lack of 'recognition' of their role, and limited authority or influence to change existing structures.

Of course, these represent worse-case scenarios, and the research found examples of good practice that not only benefited patients directly, but also empowered faith community leaders to meet patient need more effectively. For example, one hospital in the Midlands had taken the initiative of placing a small arrow on the ceiling of wards, indicating the direction of Makkah for Muslims wishing to say prayers. Some chaplaincies had made a 'calendar' of major religious festivals available to ward staff, so that they were aware of significant dates and celebrations. Additionally, over the past 12 months, at least four different hospitals have provided prayer rooms for the use of Muslim patients, recognising that facilities to pray are highly significant for the spiritual well-being of Muslim patients and their families.[12]

However, it seems to be apparent that the goodwill and theology of the senior Anglican chaplain is a significant factor in the degree of inclusion or exclusion of faith community leaders. They can exercise a good deal of influence upon whether multi-faith initiatives translate from rhetoric to reality, and whether the composition of the chaplaincy 'team' adequately reflects the religious make-up of the local community without being merely tokenism.

At present, religious community leaders who offer their time and support to hospital patients appear to be located on a blurred boundary between inclusion and exclusion. The opportunities for providing care to patients from their tradition are likely to be affected by their place on this boundary, and the degree to which their role as part of the chaplaincy team is recognised. Some faith communities are now pressing for greater recognition, and as part of this, undertaking the provision and organisation of training for their religious professionals and community leaders in pastoral care. For example, the Muslim Council of Britain now provides training, paid for by the Department of Health, for Muslims who wish to take up health care chaplaincy as a profession.[13] The NHS 'Multi-Faith Joint National Consultation' has made similar grants available to other traditions. As yet, it is too early to assess the take-up of these opportunities, and to evaluate what impact they will have for patients themselves.

This chapter has shown that the pastoral care of religious minorities reflects a range of social factors that are both internal and external to hospitals. However, as the confidence and political recognition of faith communities increases, we can expect to see the gradual evolution of more equitable arrangements for securing the spiritual welfare of patients from Britain's smaller faith traditions.

Notes

1.   Some of the themes in this chapter reflect research carried out in the Department of Sociology at the University of Warwick 1994–6, conducted by Professor James Beckford and the author. 'The Church of England and Other Faiths Project' sought to find out how effective Anglican 'brokerage' was for the inclusion of minority faith traditions in publicly funded chaplaincy (in prisons and hospitals) and in civic religion. A summary report of the research is published and available from the

Department of Sociology at Warwick University (Beckford and Gilliat 1996). See Beckford and Gilliat (1998) for a full account of the project's findings in relation to prisons.

2. I have deliberately excluded smaller or new religious movements from this chapter, though some of the issues discussed will apply to them as well as to the larger minority faith groups.

3. For a helpful overview of some major sociological trends in religious belief and practice as they apply to UK health care contexts, see Cobb and Davie (1998).

4. See Gilliat-Ray (2000) for a fuller discussion of 'approximation'.

5. To see the original advertisement, see the monthly British Muslim magazine Q News, June 2000.

6. Some of the health care chaplains who responded to the questionnaire circulated as part of the 'Church of England and Other Faiths Project', indicated their involvement in the training of nurses, though it was not a high priority.

7. There seems to be very little communication between specialist nursing academics who write about 'transcultural nursing' and those interested in spirituality. Lea's (1994) critique of cultural 'checklists' comes out of the field of transcultural nursing, and her comments suggest that effective care for patients from different world religions would be enhanced by a dialogue between nursing academics interested in spirituality, and those with expertise on transcultural nursing.

8. The research findings indicated that 47 per cent of 'Visiting Ministers' working in health care institutions regarded their access to chaplaincy records as inadequate.

9. The project discovered that one third of the Visiting Ministers from other faiths had never been in formal meetings with Anglican chaplains; evidence of Visiting Ministers' participation in genuinely multi-faith initiatives was slight (2 reports out of 26 responses).

10. Of the 26 respondents, 9 had had some involvement in training activities, but this was not extensive nor part of more methodical training programmes.

11. We found that only two of the Visiting Ministers in our sample who had access to a special room for the use of other faiths had ever been consulted about its use.

12. The *British Muslims Monthly Survey* (published by the Centre for the Study of Islam and Christian–Muslim Relations, Birmingham University) carries regular reports about the opening of prayer rooms in hospitals around the country. This figure (four in the past 12 months, from September 1999–2000) only represents provision that has been reported in national or local press; it is likely that other hospitals have made similar provision that has not been reported.

13. See the notice in *The Muslim News*, 27 October 2000, p. 11.

References

Beckford, J. and Gilliat, S. (1996) *The Church of England and Other Faiths in a Multi-faith Society.* Coventry: Department of Sociology, University of Warwick.

Beckford, J. and Gilliat, S. (1998) *Religion in Prison: Equal Rites in a Multi-faith Society.* Cambridge: Cambridge University Press.

Berthoud, R. (1997) 'Income and Standards of Living.' In T. Modood, R. Berthoud *et al.* (eds), *Ethnic Minorities in Britain: Diversity and Disadvantage.* London: Policy Studies Institute, 150–183.

Berthoud, R. and Beishon, S. (1997) 'People, Families and Households.' In T. Modood, R. Berthoud, J. Lakey, J. Nazroo, P. Smith, S. Virdee and S. Beishen (eds), *Ethnic Minorities in Britain: Diversity and Disadvantage.* London: Policy Studies Institute, 18–59.

Cobb, M. and Davie, G. (1998) 'Faith and belief: a sociological perspective.' In M. Cobb and V. Robshaw (eds) *The Spiritual Challenge of Health Care.* Edinburgh: Churchill Livingstone, 89–104.

Department of Health (1999) *The Patient's Charter.* London: HMSO

Gerrish, K. (1997) 'Preparation of nurses to meet the needs of an ethnically diverse society.' *Nurse Education Today 17,* 359–365.

Gilliat-Ray, S. (2000) *Religion in Higher Education: The Politics of the Multi-Faith Campus.* Aldershot: Ashgate.

Henley, A. and Schott, J. (1999) *Culture, Religion and Patient Care.* London: Age Concern.

Lea, A. (1994) 'Nursing in today's multicultural society: a transcultural perspective.' *Journal of Advanced Nursing 20,* 307–313.

Narayanasamy, A. (1991) *Spiritual Care: A Practical Guide for Nurses.* Lancaster: Quay Publishing.

Runnymede Trust (2000) *The Future of Multi-Ethnic Britain: The Parekh Report.* London: Runnymede Trust.

Sampson, C. (1982) *The Neglected Ethic: Religious and Cultural Factors in the Care of Patients.* London: McGraw-Hill.

Schott, J. and Henley, A. (1996) *Culture, Religion and Childbearing in a Multiracial Society.* Oxford: Butterworth Heinemann.

Walter, T. (1997) 'The ideology and organisation of pastoral care: three approaches.' *Palliative Medicine 11,* 21–30.

Weller, P. (ed) (1997) *Religions in the UK: a Multi-Faith Directory.* Derby: University of Derby/Interfaith Network for the UK.

CHAPTER 11

Being There?

Presence and Absence in Spiritual Care Delivery

Helen Orchard

The words 'being there' are common currency among spiritual care givers. The importance of being with patients and relatives can be found in the work of chaplains (Scott 2000; Speck 1988; Stoter 1995); as well as those with medical (Heyse-Moore 1996) and nursing backgrounds (Ross 1998; McSherry 2000). Wilfred McSherry, for example, suggests:

> By far the greatest consolation an individual can have when experiencing a spiritual concern is knowing that someone is there for him or her in this time of need. Presence means being with the individual in a physical and psychological sense. (p.119)

'Being there' is about providing a presence — to individual patients, to groups of staff, to the hospital as a whole community. That the provision of a presence is perceived to be an important component of spiritual care giving raises the question of what happens when there is *no* presence. A full understanding of the impact of presence surely requires a look at its flip side: absence. The full picture of spiritual care in today's NHS includes not just those who are busy being there, but also those who, for some reason, are not there at all. This chapter uses research undertaken in London hospitals as a case study for exploring the other side of being there.[1] Three straightforward questions are posed to explore the issue: Who is absent? Why are they absent? and what are the consequences of their absence?

Who is absent?

To understand the dynamics of spiritual care giving in London's hospitals, it is first necessary to outline something of the context in which this care is provided. The capital is home to more than 50 NHS Trusts,[2] providing services to a resident population of over 7 million people as well as a significant number of patients referred in from outside the Greater London area. It is the most ethnically diverse of UK cities (Storkey 1993. See also Parekh 2000). In 1999, 25 per cent of its population was made up of people from black or ethnic minority groups, with the percentage in some London boroughs estimated at 50 per cent (NHSE London 1999 and 2000). While central, reliable data sources exist on the ethnicity of the population, they are not available for religion, with ethnicity being a poor indicator of religious affiliation. Nevertheless, the spiritually cosmopolitan nature of the many parts of the capital can be evidenced by the extensive listings of its certified places of worship and community centres, affiliated to different religious groups. Weller's *Multi-Faith Directory*, for example, lists 395 Muslim, 213 Hindu, 183 Jewish and 42 Sikh organisations and worship centres in the Greater London area (1997). It is within this diverse environment that the provision of spiritual care within the health care sector must be viewed.

Table 11.1 Funded chaplaincy sessions in London's acute Trusts (1999)

Denomination	Number of sessions	Per cent
Christian		
Anglican	514	59
Roman Catholic	152	17
Free Church	153.5	18
Other	0.5	negligible
Muslim	28	3
Jewish	8	1
Hindu	0	0
Sikh	0	0
Non-specific 'minority faith'	14	2
Total	870	100

The 'official' picture of spiritual care is best represented by the number and type of funded sessions (3.5 hours) of chaplaincy time. In 1999, sessions in the acute hospital sector in London (33 Trusts) were distributed as shown in Table 11.1.

As can be seen from the table, of 870 funded chaplaincy sessions, 820 are Christian, with 514 of these Anglican. Funded sessions committed to faiths other than Christian are under 6 per cent, with no funded sessions at all allocated to six of Britain's nine major faith groups. Translating sessions into actual care givers to provide an indication of the composition of chaplaincy teams alters the overall picture very little, as can be seen from Table 11.2.

Table 11.2 Chaplaincy team composition in London's acute Trusts (Headcount in 1999)			
Denomination	Paid staff	Visiting ministers	Volunteers
Christian			
Anglican	68	23	152
Roman Catholic	57	17	129
Free Church	37	6	58
Other	0	2	36
Muslim	8	5	14
Jewish	8	17	53
Hindu	0	0	6
Sikh	0	0	2
Non-specific 'minority faith'	1	0	0
Total	179	70	450

While staffing figures in this table are no surprise given the distribution of funded sessions, it is interesting that for non-funded positions, such as volunteers and visiting ministers, the presence of minority faiths is also sparse. There are no official visiting ministers in acute London Trusts for Hindus and Sikhs and the number of volunteers from these faith groups is also low: six Hindus (from three Trusts) and two Sikhs (from one Trust). In addition, sizeable proportions of chaplaincies in London appear to have no contact at all with a Muslim or Jewish representative (with the percentages being 55 per cent and 30 per cent respectively). The other four religions which are generally included within the list of the UK's nine major faith groups (Buddhists, Baha'is, Jains and Zoroastrians) do not appear at all.

Such statistics on minority faith representation are unlikely to surprise those working in the field, but this level of absence is nevertheless notable, particularly given the length of time the service has had to make progress toward the implementation of official NHS guidance on the matter. Despite the exhortations of Health Service Guideline 92(2) that Trusts should 'recognise the welfare needs of both Christians and non Christians', deciding how to provide services 'after consulting their local community' (NHSME 1992, p.1), there still seems to be little by way of collaboration between chaplaincies and local faith leaders. This is borne out by the London research, which reveals a significant gap between the aspirations and praxis of chaplains. When asked about the challenges facing their service in a questionnaire, multi-faith collaboration was the most frequently mentioned issue, with over 70 per cent of all respondents making reference to it. Despite this, only nine departments in the whole of the London region had a mechanism in place for liaising with faith leaders in the community through, for example, a multi-cultural forum or faith and health group. Informal networking practices were similarly under-developed: when asked how official representatives of faith communities were selected for the Trust, only 35 per cent of departments were using networking and informal contacts with local faith communities. Three chaplaincies said they *did not know* how representatives were selected (Orchard 2000, p.38).

Why are they absent?

There are clearly numerous, composite reasons underpinning the minority faith absence in this area of health care: funding and resourcing issues, theology and churchmanship, organisational and practical reasons, politics and prejudice. The answer lies in a combination of many of these. At the risk of over-simplifying, this section simply selects the four most prevalent themes that emerged from the London research as reasons for the under-representation of minority faiths to explore in brief: the financial pretext, the brokerage pretext, the complexity pretext and the 'unnatural act' pretext.

The financial pretext

While funding is an obvious contributing factor, it did not appear to be the primary reason for the lack of minority faith presence. In the first instance it is evident that even informal mechanisms for securing inclusion within chaplaincy teams have not occurred. While the development of community contacts and input from visiting ministers or volunteers requires time and effort, it does not necessarily need much by way of budgetary increases. Funding was not essential for securing a basic level of presence within a team, but rather an official sessional presence. However, it was clear that even when funding is available, there may be other obstacles to recruitment. Several Trusts encountered in the course of the research had held monies specifically for this purpose in their budget for quite some time but had not determined how to put it to use. The argument that lack of funding is the principal obstacle to more balanced teams does not seem particularly justifiable.

The brokerage pretext

The concept of brokerage requires some explanation. What is meant by the term is the tendency of Christian chaplains, particularly Anglicans, to assume the role of a spiritual broker on behalf of all faiths, in addition to representing their own. The following quote from an Anglican chaplain makes reference to precisely this situation:

> I think that one of the things that chaplaincy could be is an honest broker in a pluralistic society... Someone has to take on the role of being an honest broker and has to be perceived as being as fair as you can be. Well I think that is something chaplains and chaplaincy departments can do if they have the courage to do it... And I think in Anglicanism there is a spirit of fairness and justice that is not in other denominations.

It is the last sentence which gives an indication of one of the problems with this approach. This chaplain has a rather exclusive attitude towards brokering care, feeling that, actually, the role of broker is best confined to Anglicans, who are able to behave in a way that others are not. A further allusion to brokerage can be seen in the comment of another chaplain:

> If you are a priest of the Church of England...you know you don't have a responsibility to minister to a believing, gathered congregation. You know that you have a responsibility to represent something for the people

who may be right outside…to make sure spiritual care is given. I think historically the Church of England, because of the establishment bit, in sometimes a kind of loose way holds on to the spiritual bit… Now I'm not sure that will always remain the same, I'm sure it's changing, but I think it's a useful role to have.

Here 'establishment' is used to justify Anglican purchase of the spiritual care of everyone. Anglicans 'hold on to' the spiritual bit, 'making sure it is given', even to those 'right outside'. In these examples we can start to glimpse the contribution brokerage makes to absence through the assumptions people adopt. If the only fit brokers are Anglicans, who by virtue of establishment 'hold on to' everyone's 'spiritual bit', it does raise questions about the role of others and even the extent to which they are needed.

This, then, is the point: brokerage has a subtle impact on the development of *formal* mechanisms for including others in the team. It diminishes an awareness of the need for religious leaders from other traditions, as the broker oversees meeting the needs of all. This does not imply that all brokerage arrangements are inherently wrong: local context is an important factor and they are inevitable to some extent for practical reasons. But the greater the diversity of the hospital population, the more problematic this model becomes. The risk is that brokerage can be patronising, exclusive and have a negative impact on the formal presence of minority faiths in the structure of the service.

The complexity pretext

The third issue – that of complexity – is linked to brokerage in some ways. The beauty of a brokerage mechanism is its ease of management: lines of accountability are very clear and recruitment is relatively straightforward. Conversely, when it comes to formally building-in minority faith representation to the structure of the chaplaincy service, it is perceived as difficult and impractical. This is a further reason for absence. The perceived difficulties cluster around two areas: the size of minority communities and the legitimacy of their leaders; and concerns over how to maintain service standards, particularly with respect to confidentiality.

It was felt by a number of chaplains interviewed that it was simply not possible to allocate sessions, or even representative status, to faiths where there was a small percentage of patients in the hospital. Moreover that committing sessions did not recognise the different organisational features of minority faiths, many of which have no centralised hierarchies acting as licensing bodies. The problem becomes one of identifying a person who can function as an 'appropriate' representative of the relevant faith community, as indicated by this comment, made by one senior chaplain:

> The way other faiths organise themselves is done locally round local temples or mosques and therefore it is sometimes difficult to know who is representative in a sense…and whether you're simply getting the person who shouted the loudest they wanted to come in and so I'm a bit wary of that sometimes.

The relative youth of ethnic minority communities is a common theme with the perception that people within them do not have, in the words of one chaplain, sufficient 'maturity of experience' to fulfil visiting roles. Allied to this is the subject of confidentiality. Several chaplains expressed the opinion that the minority faith communities, or even Christians from other cultural backgrounds, 'didn't understand' the rules of confidentiality within a hospital setting. Their involvement in care giving was consequently seen as difficult and risky, potentially exposing patients who did not want members of their community to know they were in hospital or the nature of their condition.

The 'unnatural act' pretext

Finally in this section, a further explanation for the absence of minority faiths within formal chaplaincy structures is the perception that 'being there' is something of an unnatural act for particular religions. Pastoral visiting is judged to be an alien concept, not naturally part of their culture and history, as indicated by this comment from an Anglican chaplain:

> The pattern of hospital ministry is a western European model of doing ministry, and pastoral practice is defined in that way. Minority faiths are also moving towards more western models of pastoral care, but really a rabbi is a teacher and so is an imam. Do such figures really work in such a way that they can be fitted into a sessional basis? You have to ask what are they there for?

Here, the chaplain doubts the need to allocate sessions to minority faith representatives in the way they would be to Christian chaplains, with the question 'what are they there for?' The 'being there' model of care is felt to be imposed inappropriately on patients from minority religious communities, who actually have no expectation of this kind of service at all.

The argument is: they won't notice the absence because they don't expect a presence. Moreover, there is a concern that applying the same method of sessional allocation to all chaplains and expecting the same activities from those sessions forces everyone into the Western European model, regardless of whether it is appropriate. This influence of Christian chaplaincy on the understanding of pastoral care and practice held by non-Christian religions is discussed in detail by Sophie Gilliat-Ray in Chapter 10. The point being made here is simply that the perception of this phenomenon by some chaplains functions as a further explanation for the absence of minority faith representatives from the picture.

This section has established some basic facts around who is present and absent within the structures of hospital chaplaincy, as well as exploring specific reasons. The lack of formal frameworks for providing minority faith patients with care from their own religious representatives reveals a basic structural inequity within London services. The next section discusses the implications of this inequity.

What happens in their absence?

At its most basic level, such *structural inequity* results in a *lack of choice* for minority faith patients and relatives over a suitable care giver. In the absence of such a care giver, the rites and responsibilities of another faith may be *appropriated* and delivered by the Christian chaplain. These three terms are inter-linked. *Structural inequity* results in *lack of choice* which may lead to *appropriation*. Appropriation can take a number of forms. The most common example encountered in the London research was the practice of Christian chaplains to undertake funerals for patients of other faiths – Hindu, Muslim and Jewish. While these funerals did not appear to be overly Christianised, with care being taken either to use the relevant text or to focus on humanist themes such as dignity and respect, it would perhaps not have been that surprising if they were as, astoundingly, the current official advice to Anglican chaplains remains that the form of service for these funerals 'should celebrate the Christian faith and its affirmation of the Easter victory', although 'it may be possible also to include something from the person's own tradition' (HCC 1993, p.13). Appropriation may be undertaken unwittingly and for the best of motives, but in the context of advice such as this, it is hardly surprising that it sometimes oversteps the mark. Just such a situation is revealed in this quote from an interview with a rabbi:

Rabbi:	I think there's quite a challenge...for the churches who have to learn when *not* to do things. I mean in one of my hospitals I have the most delightful Free Church chaplain. He doesn't tell me there are Jews there, he just tells me when I next bump into him that he's baptised this one, or done this one, or done that one.
Interviewer:	To the Jews?
Rabbi:	Yeah, well he said they accepted the oil and I think: *what have they accepted the oil for?* And I know what he's done, he's tried to be inclusive...and I've looked after Muslim prisoners because there was no Muslim, but I was also prepared to say that it was not appropriate and ultimately they needed a Muslim.

While this rabbi interprets the chaplain's actions rather charitably in terms of inclusivity, others may feel it borders on proselytising behaviour and it is certainly an example of a brokerage attitude that has resulted in appropriation. Christian chaplains may well feel they are in a position, as hospital representatives, to offer religious rites to all-comers and it may be entirely appropriate for them to do so, particularly if a relationship has been built up with the patient or relatives. But the underlying issue is that patients and relatives have built up a relationship with the Christian chaplain because, in all likelihood, there was no representative of their own faith made available to assist them at their time of need. The fact that a Hindu asks a Christian chaplain to undertake a funeral should not obscure the point that the service infrastructure did not provide him or her with a proper *choice* of care giver in the first place.

Some of the issues raised by appropriation are further demonstrated in the case study below, which is a section from an interview with another Christian chaplain. The chaplain was approached by a Muslim couple concerning the burial of their pre–24 week foetus. S/he explains:

They had wanted a member of their community to do some form of service..., and could not arrange that because no one could offer anything and they then came back to me and said; 'well, what do you do, what do you say?'...and I talked through what I would do and what might be possible... We agreed together how we would say some of the same sort of words but remove the Christian elements and then what we would use from their holy book... [The father] didn't feel physically able to take the coffin, put it in the ground and say his prayer. So I offered him a framework with my presence, to enable him to do that. And they were deeply appreciative and that was again one of those moments that you have sometimes when you think, yes, I happen to be a [Free Church] minister, but I was being in a true sense a hospital chaplain. But for him and me it took an awful lot of time and energy and space and commitment to reach the point of the funeral. Because we did have a tricky beginning – one conversation when I had to ring him to say 'you've filled the form in and it says Muslim, and this is what the hospital can offer', to try and tease out what they were about. He was quite sharp on the phone and not quite sure what I was really saying. So you have to be so tentative and careful.

This is clearly a complex case, which contains issues for the Muslim community as well as Christian chaplaincy. The chaplain acts in a sensitive and skilful manner, negotiating a solution which the family greatly value. While some chaplains would have declined to undertake such a ceremony, there are many others who would have taken the same action, regarding it as an example of flexible working practice in a situation where there is an absence of input from the community. However, it is also possible to examine this case using the terms introduced above: structural inequity, lack of choice and appropriation.

Structural inequity

There was no Muslim chaplain, visiting minister or formal arrangement in this Trust for providing Muslim patients with a core element of NHS care. Interestingly, the department did have links with a surgeon who acted as an informal Muslim adviser on occasion. But when the chaplain was asked whether contact would be made with him in this sort of situation, the response was: 'It's an interesting question, we've not explored that area.' The result is that 'what the hospital has to offer' is limited to what can be delivered by the default position of the Christian chaplain. This is not conscious or deliberate exclusion, it is an inevitable consequence of the way the service is configured.

Absence of choice

The family wanted someone from their own faith to help them with this traumatic event. They got a service but it wasn't the service they would have chosen had there been an alternative. The point here is not whether an imam would have handled the situation in a similar way, or actually whether any ceremony would have been provided at all. The point is that the structural inequity within the chaplaincy service meant the religious and cultural preferences of the family could not be respected by the hospital. Instead, it was a case of making the best of what was on offer, which actually made things more difficult for them at an already difficult time.

Appropriation

What happens in a situation of appropriation is that a substitute presence is provided by a Christian chaplain. The type of presence requested and needed by the patient is not available. The broker steps into the gap in the service and uses his or her own presence to provide what is required. In this case, the chaplain even uses the words, saying: 'I offered him a framework with *my presence*...to enable him to do that.' The real question is what the chaplain's responsibility is in this sort of situation. Is it to broker a solution by someone of the relevant faith, or is it to take that step, providing the solution personally? This is a complex question, meriting serious debate by the profession.

Concluding comment

This chapter has taken an alternative approach to the concept of presence to discuss one aspect of spiritual care services. It has revealed who is absent from London's chaplaincy services, posited reasons for their absence and explored the consequences in terms of the provision of substitute presence. It is important to make clear that the absence of minority faith groups from the structure of services is not a situation created or perpetuated deliberately. The little research and writing there is on this subject has revealed that in general, chaplains aspire to be more inclusive in their practices (Beckford and Gilliat 1996; Olumide 1993). The significant delay in translating these aspirations into a practical reality has no doubt been exacerbated by a lack of proactive leadership on this matter at a national level (Orchard 2000). To achieve that translation, a far more sustained engagement with local communities will be needed, together with a greater commitment to creative ways of formally including people. This would involve developing mechanisms of recognising the status of individuals as qualified and competent representatives, agreeing appropriate remuneration, according rights of access and sharing power and decision making. Securing the presence of those currently absent in a way that is practical, manageable and makes sense for the communities concerned will be no mean feat. It is, however, essential if patients and staff are to be cared for in ways that genuinely meet their needs on their own terms.

Notes

1. The research was undertaken in London in 1999 and funded by The King's Fund. All quotes from chaplains included in this chapter are taken from taped interviews which formed part of the fieldwork.

2. At the time of writing, there were 57 Trusts in London, although the numbers are in a continuous state of flux as rationalisation and reorganisation of hospital sites and structures takes place.

References

Beckford, J. A. and Gilliat, S. (1996) *The Church of England and other Faiths in a Multi-Faith Society.* Warwick Working Papers in Sociology 21. Warwick: University of Warwick.

Heyse-Moore, L. H. (1996) 'On spiritual pain in the dying.' *Mortality 1*, 3, 297–315.

Hospital Chaplaincies Council (1993) *Our Ministry and Other Faiths: A Booklet for Hospital Chaplains.* 2nd edn; London: Central Board of Finance for the Church of England.

McSherry, W. (2000) *Making Sense of Spirituality in Nursing Practice.* Edinburgh: Churchill Livingstone.

NHSE London (1999) 'Health and ethnicity in London.' Unpublished paper of the NHSE London.

NHSE London (2000) *The London Health Strategy.* London: Department of Health.

NHSME (1992) 'Meeting the spiritual needs of patients and staff.' Health Service Guideline 92(2).

Olumide, O. (1993) Towards equitable provision of spiritual, religious and cultural care within the NHS.' *Journal of Health Care Chaplaincy*, Sept 1993, 12–16.

Orchard, H. (2000) *Hospital Chaplaincy: Modern, Dependable?* Sheffield: Sheffield Academic Press.

Parekh, B. (chair) (2000) *The Future of Multi-Ethnic Britain.* London: Profile Books.

Ross, L. (1998) 'The nurse's role in spiritual care.' In M. Cobb and V. Robshaw (eds) *The Spiritual Challenge of Health Care.* Edinburgh: Churchill Livingstone.

Scott, T. (2000) 'Chaplaincy – a resource of Christian presence.' *Scottish Journal of Health care Chaplaincy 3*, 1, 15–19.

Speck, P.W. (1988) *Being There: Pastoral Care in Time of Illness.* London: SPCK.

Storkey, M. (1993) *London's Ethnic Minorities: One City, Many Communities*. London: London Research Centre.

Stoter, D. (1995) *Spiritual Aspects of Health Care*. London: Mosby.

Weller, P. (ed) (1997) *Religions in the UK: A Multi-Faith Directory*. Derby: University of Derby and The Inter Faith Network.

CHAPTER 12

Jewish Spirituality
The Impact on Health Care

Martin van den Bergh

Judaism promotes the care of the sick as a supreme religious act. It has always understood the importance of a holistic approach to patient care, for humans are not merely physical beings, they also have a spiritual entity. Therefore when the body is afflicted by a physical ailment, its spiritual essence also suffers. We may think that 'spirituality' no longer has any place in today's increasingly secularised society. Yet even though the influence of organised religion may have diminished, there is still spiritual searching and a need for a spiritual meaning to life. These needs are especially emphasised when we are confronted with life crises, or our human fallibility is highlighted. When our whole concept of life is challenged, our spiritual concerns spring to the fore. Even those who may not describe themselves as being 'religious' or spiritually inclined will usually turn to their own faith traditions to find a response to their spiritual needs.

How does Judaism respond to these spiritual needs? It may be difficult to understand how it can respond. The problem arises in finding a Jewish definition of 'spirituality', and in understanding whether there is a Jewish pastoral theology that is sensitive to the needs of patients. In a modern health care environment, where clearly defined workable definitions are needed, overcoming such difficulties is important if the spiritual needs of patients who require a Jewish response are to be met.

Aspects of Jewish spirituality

Judaism is a faith system that lives its spirituality rather than pondering on what it really means. This is a vital component of its religious make-up and is

160

derived theologically from the Old Testament teaching that man is created in the image of God. Rabbi Aaron Twersky, in his foreword to *Medicine in the Mishnei Torah of Maimonides*, says that man was created both as a spiritual and a physical being.[1] Therefore 'the reality of man's existence is not physical but spiritual' (Rosner 1984, p.xii). This is based on teaching found in the Book of Ecclesiastes 12:7: 'And the dust returns to the earth as it was; and the spirit returns to God who gave it.'

Chief Rabbi Sacks (1995) explains that Jewish spirituality has been the very essence of Jewish survival. It has survived many national calamities through its long history. The classic work that echoes this is the Book of Job, and the Talmud goes so far as to say that true spirituality can only be achieved by trials and tribulations. Rabbi Harold Kushner (1982) echoes this theory by relating his own experiences of losing a son through illness. Rabbi Dr Abraham Twersky states that 'spirituality can be seen as being synonymous with humanity', namely it describes those traits that separate humans from animals. These traits give humanity the capacity to learn from the past; to think about the goal and purpose of existence; to self-improve; to delay gratification; to reflect on the consequences of actions; to control anger; to forgive; and ultimately 'to be free'(Twersky 1998, p.18).

Arthur Green defines spirituality as: 'Life in the presence of God or the cultivation of a life in the ordinary world bearing the holiness once associated with sacred space and time, with Temple and with holy days.' Echoing the difficulty of coming to a precise definition, he admits this description 'is perhaps as close as one can come to a definition of spirituality that is native to the Jewish tradition and indeed faithful to its Semitic roots' (1987, p.xii).

Jewish spirituality impacts upon our daily lives as an expression of the command 'you shall be holy' (Lev. 11:45), and as a part of our obligation to emulate God's attributes of mercy and compassion. The command to be holy is reflected in the dietary laws, the keeping of the Sabbath laws, our laws of marriage and family, and our behaviour towards our fellow man. It is the continual endeavour to turn the mundane into something sacred or 'spiritual'. This can best be illustrated by the Jewish tradition of saying a blessing before partaking of food. This simple act does not only fulfil the requirement of thanking God for all our sustenance; it turns a simple and physical act of taking nourishment into a sacred act. The obligation to emulate God's attributes is reflected in our duty to be compassionate, merciful and forgiving; to visit and care for the sick, the disadvantaged; and to rehabilitate the sinner. Therefore our spirituality becomes in a sense second nature – we do not even dwell or think about it; we live it.

Translating Jewish spirituality into the health care environment

Living one's spirituality may be a good way of answering spiritual needs. However, there are inherent difficulties, both for the religiously observant and for the not-so-religious Jewish patient. Both will still have spiritual needs. The observant Jewish patient will rightly want to observe his or her faith as much as possible in a health care environment through rituals of the faith. Observance in itself will be a source of spiritual comfort. However, it should not be assumed that this will address all the patient's needs. The non-observant Jewish patient may find greater difficulty in discovering his or her spiritual needs in a ritual that has been neglected or rejected, and thus the ability to express one's spirituality has also been lost. Yet the Jewish patient may still turn to Judaism for spiritual comfort and support. Laurence J. Silbertstein suggests how to respond to the Jew who has been alienated from the faith at a time of spiritual need: 'The task of the religious teacher is not to induct persons into a system of observances and teachings, but to awaken their sense of awe and wonder' (1987, p.402).

Experience has shown that spiritual needs are not limited to observant Jews. In the context of health care, possibly the call for greater spiritual care is demanded from those less identified with the Jewish community. Such Jews may indeed suffer greater spiritual stress at times of crisis. First, because they feel less able to find expression for their spiritual needs – for example, they are less able to pray. Second, this may produce more frustration or feelings of shame. In such cases any assessment of spiritual needs will have to be more sensitive when identifying such concerns. In addition, careful consideration has to be given to the provision of those spiritual needs. In some cases it is appropriate for a Jewish chaplain or minister of religion to be called, in order for a process of reconciliation to be undertaken. In other cases it would be more appropriate for the Jewish chaplain not to be called if it would cause more anxiety. In some cases the administration of spiritual care to Jewish patients can be dispensed by a Jewish lay visitor who can act as a bridge with the community that the patient may feel alienated from, yet may feel a need for at least some contact with his or her Jewish roots. An understanding of Jewish spiritual needs is complicated not only by the difficulty in defining *what* Jewish spirituality is, but also by the difficulty of *how* to recognise the needs.

The transfer of spiritual identity from a more social and communal base to a personal need brings it into the realm of personal privacy. Unless the patient is willing to enunciate his or her innermost feelings, any spiritual needs assessment cannot be accomplished. The assessor, whether a nurse or a chaplain, has first to secure the confidence of the patient. The reserved nature of British culture means we may hesitate to probe too readily into somebody else's private thoughts, preferring to dwell on the trivia: 'How are you, how is the weather, and what did you see on the TV last night?' We may even permit ourselves to engage in some religious activity as a means of mechanical action, rather than expressing deeper thoughts or feelings. In the USA, experience of hospital visiting reveals a people far more open, making it easier to 'probe' deeper into the minds of others who are more 'up front' about their inner thoughts. In a Jewish context this is further assisted by the fact that even though patients or their families may have forsaken their religious identity as Jews, they still retain their cultural identity as Jews and are therefore able to express spiritual requirements in this way.

Most faith traditions have a well-established system of addressing life crises, drawing upon particular scriptures, traditions and interpretations, to find meaning in the face of adversity. Judaism, like many other doctrinal faiths, answers these dilemmas within well-defined parameters. Those who may not subscribe to such an approach will contend that such a doctrinal approach has no place today in a pastoral setting. They find it difficult to comprehend how these methods can adequately address certain scenarios people have to contend with, either as individuals, as a part of a community or as a part of society in general. One of the reasons for this perception is the view that there is a conflict between theological perspectives and pastoral necessities. Christians have attempted to resolve this by developing a pastoral theology which takes as its starting point the situation or the patient, and works from there to resolve inconsistencies in what is termed 'The Hebrew Bible' and other classical theological works. Orthodox Judaism, which is built upon the authenticity and divine authority of its scriptures, has to find another way to resolve this conflict, if it can at all. This brings us to the question of whether there is a Jewish pastoral theology. Are there conflicts between upholding Jewish doctrine, while trying to give maximum spiritual and pastoral care? Is it possible to resolve these conflicts?

Is there a Jewish pastoral theology?

Joseph Ozarwoski gives a strong affirmative answer to this question. He defines Jewish pastoral care as: 'using the tools of Jewish tradition, liturgy, and philosophy to guide people though crisis periods'. He believes that 'Jewish tradition offers great therapeutic benefit to those in these painful situations' (Ozarwoski 1995, p.11). The basis of this theology is the Hebrew Bible. Orthodox Judaism interprets the Bible using a very distinct set of rules, termed 'The Oral Tradition', which was first set out by the sages of the Talmud, and continues to this day. Other writers disagree with the conclusions of Ozarowski. Deborah van Deusen Hunsinger, for example, focuses on what she feels are inconsistencies in the theology of the Hebrew Bible which describes God as being compassionate and just, yet also presents God as destructive and insensitive to the vulnerable (van Deusen Hunsinger 1995). She illustrates the apparent insensitivity to rape and violence against women, by highlighting the stories of Hagar and the rape of Tamar. This seems to give the impression that there is very wide gap between Jewish theology and matters of pastoral care.

Orthodox Judaism however sees no conflict between the two. Its scriptures promote an all-embracing way of life based upon the teachings of the Torah (The Five Books of Moses) as interpreted by rabbinical tradition. Rabbinic tradition is expounded mainly in the Babylonian Talmud and in the codification of Jewish Law by Rabbi Joseph Caro, called the *Shulchan Aruch*.[2] Ozarowski notes that Judaism teaches us that 'we affirm life even while facing pain and death' (1995, p.3). Holding these two elements in tension enables us to use Jewish theology as a basis for pastoral care. This is accomplished by imitating our Creator – walking in God's paths – and through acts of loving-kindness. Ozarowski supports this claim from the Talmud:

> What does it mean: 'You shall walk after the Lord your God'? (Deuteronomy 13.5). Is it, then, possible for a human being to walk and follow God's presence? For has it not been said: 'For the Lord your God is a consuming fire'? (Deuteronomy 4.24). But it means to walk after the attributes of the Holy One, blessed be He. Just as He clothes the naked, for it is written: 'And the Lord God made for Adam and for his wife coats of skin, and clothed them,' (Genesis 3.21) so you too clothe the naked. The Holy One, blessed be He, visited the sick, for it is written: 'And the Lord appeared unto him by the oaks of Mamre' (Genesis 18.1), so you too shall visit the sick. The Holy One, blessed be He, comforted mourners, for it is

written: 'And it came to pass after the death of Abraham, that God blessed Isaac his son' (Genesis 25.11), so too shall you comfort the bereaved. The Holy one, blessed be He, buried the dead, for it is written: 'And He buried him in the valley' (Deuteronomy 34.6), so you too bury the dead. (Babylonian Talmud. Tractate Sotah 14a)

Ozarowski draws on another Talmudic source to illustrate the notion that we can walk in God's ways not only by observing the rituals (such as keeping the dietary laws and the Sabbath), but also by 'connecting to each other and caring for each other, specifically at moments of illness and grief' (1995, p.4). As the Babylonian Talmud establishes:

These are the things of which one enjoys the fruits in this world, while the principle remains in the hereafter, namely – honouring father and mother; the practice of kindness; early attendance at the house of study morning and evening; hospitality to strangers; visiting the sick; dowering the bride; attending the dead; devotion in prayer; making peace between people.' (Babylonian Talmud. Tractate Shabbat 127a)

Despite evidence to support the argument that Jewish pastoral theology is imbedded within the traditional sources of Judaism, there is a mistaken view that Orthodox Jewish theology cannot meet pastoral needs. Even those who may not subscribe to an Orthodox Jewish approach, will acknowledge the link between the Hebrew Bible and pastoral care. Harold Kushner, a conservative rabbi argues that 'there is a straight line from the biblical story of the Exodus to contemporary Jewish involvement in issues of social justice'. He adds that ritual re-emphasises this: 'remembering, and annually repeating, the story of slavery and liberation (the observance of the Passover), we have developed a sense of empathy for the oppressed' (Kushner 1993, p.45). Pastoral care within Judaism is an integral part of its theology: Jewish pastoral theology is not a separate entity. Yet, even though its sources promote pastoral care, does Judaism not suffer from the same difficulty as any dogmatic system; unable to be sensitive and flexible to pastoral needs?

Is Jewish law sensitive to pastoral needs?

A closer look at the laws of visiting the sick, included in the *Shulchan Aruch*, reveals their sensitivity to the needs of patients. Even though visiting the sick is considered to be a most meritorious act, it nevertheless should not be undertaken if it causes greater anxiety to the patient. For example, the sick should not be visited in the first and last three hours of the day and visiting should not be undertaken to those suffering from intestinal disorders, eye disease or diseases of the head. In addition, the act of visiting should be undertaken in such a way as will maintain the dignity of the patient because, as Ozarowski cites, 'God's presence is above the patient's head' (1995, p.4).[3] He further suggests that Judaism does not only promote pastoral care, it emphasises the importance of sensitive and empathetic delivery, commenting that 'the giver's understanding and conveying that understanding to the sufferer help alleviate the sense of loneliness and thus alleviate the pain itself' (p.22). It is understandable for this sensitivity to be present when the sufferer may still subscribe to the same theology (even though his incapacity may cause his non-observance of certain Jewish laws) as Jewish law allows for this. However, is it possible to empathise with someone who rejects, or who is at a variance with, Jewish dogma? The answer may lie in examining the Jewish approach to repentance and salvation.

The Jewish approach to repentance and salvation

One of the most important functions of pastoral care is to provide a mechanism by which the patient or client can find peace of mind. There is a need for an affirmation of life and reconciliation, both with God and one's neighbour, particularly in life-threatening situations. The process of repentance in Jewish theology is designed to achieve this goal. It is not intended to be judgmental; rather a way of bringing a transgressor to a realisation of the folly of his or her ways. It provides an opportunity to resolve the conflicts that exist within him or herself, and with those who have been offended, both God and man.

The 12th-century rabbi Moses Maimonides in his epic work *Mishnei Torah* gives a very clear set of guidelines to achieve reconciliation through the act of repentance (Maimonides' Laws of Repentance 3:14). An insight into this procedure shows that Maimonides was not only explaining the laws, but also revealing the psychology behind them. There is a clear biblical command to repent: 'And you shall return and obey the voice of the Lord, and do all his commandments which I command you this day' (Deut. 30:8). The Hebrew Bible recognises that 'there is not a just man upon earth, that does good, and does not sin' (Eccles. 7:20). Although repentance is more relevant for the Day of Atonement, Maimonides states that one can repent at any time. Central to the process of repentance is the acknowledgement of transgression of sins, which is accomplished by the utterance of a confessional prayer. In a pastoral context, a person can say a similar confessional prayer on the verge of death. Experience has shown that in cases where such a prayer can be administered to a terminal patient, it can achieve a great sense of tranquillity and peace of mind.

Maimonides writes: 'Even if a person denies God's existence throughout his life and repents in his final moments, he merits a portion in the world to come' (Maimonides Laws of Repentance 3:14). The gates of repentance are always open as the Prophet Isaiah says: '"Peace, peace, to the distant and the near" declares God. "I will heal him"' (Isa. 57:19). This review of the Orthodox Jewish approach to repentance and salvation gives a very clear indicator of how Jewish dogma promotes a pastoral concern that is not judgmental and that is sensitive. It provides for a six-point process of salvation: admission of guilt/confession; repentance; judgement; atonement/punishment; reconciliation; and, finally, peace of mind. Yet can this sensitivity exist when there are demands by the patient or the patient's family, that contravene Jewish law, such as euthanasia or cremation?

Sensitivity in difficult situations

Orthodox Judaism, which retains a strict adherence to Jewish law, finds it difficult, yet not impossible, to address obscure situations. Progressive Judaism, although subscribing to Jewish biblical scriptures, rejects strict interpretation of Jewish law, and therefore has no difficulty in addressing such situations. How can Orthodox Judaism address these situations without abrogating its laws?

Ozarowski discusses the issue of comforting a family of a 37-year-old man who was cremated. Jewish tradition is strongly opposed to cremation. Jewish law does not normally permit the ashes to be interred in a Jewish cemetery, or for mourning practices to be observed for the deceased. However, in some London Jewish Orthodox communities, the burial of ashes is permitted within certain conditions. Ozarowski reflects on how he wanted to offer comfort and support the parents in coming to terms with their loss, while maintaining his halachic (Jewish law) standards and integrity as an orthodox rabbi. He found a way to fulfil his pastoral function of enabling his family to grieve in a way consistent with Jewish tradition. The basis of his approach was a rabbinical source which states: 'But for what applies to honour for the living, Rabbi Hazan in *Hayyei Olam*[4] allows us to comfort the mourners for a cremated person' (Kol Bo 21:53–54). This source is also used to support the lenient approach taken in the case of suicide. Jewish law also takes a very strong stand against suicide, yet will permit the utmost leniency in comforting the mourners. Most rabbinical authorities will also tend to be lenient in permitting the burial of a suicide in the normal way so as not to cause greater suffering to the mourners, although this contradicts strict Jewish law.

Although Orthodox Judaism may appear to be an unbending dogmatic faith, it provides a code to be lived in the real world. It recognises the world with all its imperfections, and therefore is able to confront modern dilemmas. John Patton comments, 'it is in the world that we find God' (1990). The Hebrew Bible is full of inconsistencies because humanity is full of inconsistencies. It even portrays its personalities as people who are not infallible. Rabbinic sources are able to draw upon Jewish theology in order to confront the challenges life brings. While promoting a strict dogma, it is therefore also able to be sensitive to pastoral needs. Judaism is able to be responsive not only in life-threatening situations, but also in other crisis scenarios. Is it possible to conclude that there is no conflict between Jewish dogma and practice in pastoral care?

Is there a conflict between Jewish dogma and practice in pastoral care?

I have attempted to show that Judaism does not see a need for a separate discipline of pastoral theology. It can also be argued that Jewish sources, traditions and codes provide for sensitive and empathetic consideration in all situations. Even when Jewish law has been breached, there is room for providing support. However, this relies on two important assumptions. First, that the providers of pastoral and spiritual care fully understand that their role in a theological sense is to emulate God's attributes of mercy and compassion. Their role is not to force the strict adherence of Jewish dogma, while not transgressing it or abetting its infringement. Second, that those who are vulnerable will not become victims to those who have other agendas, and will be caused greater harm and anxiety.

In my experience, the two assumptions are not always upheld. A fundamentalist would find it hard not to bring into a pastoral situation other issues. For example, a discussion with a ministerial colleague on the purpose of visiting the sick revealed his main aim was to ensure the patient has kosher meals. My response to him was that, if the patient wants kosher meals, *only then* is it our duty to ensure that there is provision for such meals. If the aim is to force dogma, then that aim is incompatible with pastoral care.

Conclusions

An examination of traditional Jewish theological sources, both biblical and rabbinic, shows that Jewish dogma can be responsive to crisis situations, and one can find meaning in the face of adversity. However, for a chaplain or any other care giver to be effective in a pastoral environment an empathetic approach needs to be established so that he or she is not only ministering out of a sense of duty, but from a real sense of caring. Even though the care giver may subscribe to a well-defined and established faith tradition, that same background should impress the need not to be judgmental. A Jewish chaplain's training will teach him at least to respect the person as a fellow human being made in the image of God. Jewish doctrine does provide a mechanism to resolve most points of conflict between dogma and practice, especially in pastoral situations. Even when these conflicts cannot be resolved, the care giver can still have compassion and stand alongside those who are suffering, without necessarily contravening Jewish theology.

Notes

1. *Mishnei Torah* is the opus magnum of Rabbi Moses Maimonides, who was born in Cordova, Spain in 1135. He was a rabbi and the spiritual leader of the Jewish community of Egypt. He was the personal physician to Vizier Al Fadhil, regent of Egypt during the absence of the Sultan, Saladin the Great, who fought in the Crusades in Palestine.

2. The *Shulchan Aruch* was compiled by Rabbi Joseph Caro, a 16th-century scholar, and was added to by the 16th-century Rabbi Moses Isserles to make it applicable to the whole of World Jewry. It is the codification of Jewish Law, which is still recognised as the guide of Orthodox Jewry to this day.

3. Ozarwoski summarises the laws of visiting the sick in the appendix of his book 'To walk in God's Ways'.

4. The *Hayyei Olam* is a pre-modern Hebrew work on mourning.

References

Babylonion Talmud. Sotah 14a and Shabbat 127a. Brooklyn, NY: Judaica Press, Inc. 1990 (CD-ROM edition).

Green, A. (ed) (1987) *Jewish Spirituality.* Vol. I, London: SCM Press.

Kushner, H. (1982) *When Bad Things Happen to Good People.* London: Pan Books.

Kushner, H. (1993) *To Life: A Celebration of Jewish Being and Thinking.* London: Little, Brown and Company.

Ozarwoski, J. S. (1995) *To Walk in God's Ways: Jewish Pastoral Perspectives on Illness and Bereavement.* Northvale, New Jersey: Aronson.

Patton, J. (1990) *Ministry for Theology: Pastoral Action and Reflection.* Nashville: Abingdon.

Rosner, F. (1984) *Medicine in the Mishnei Torah of Maimonides.* Ktav Publishing House.

Sacks, J. (1995) *Faith in the Future.* London: Darton, Longman and Todd.

Silbertstein, L. (1987) 'The renewal of Jewish Spirituality: two views.' In A. Green (ed) *Jewish Spirituality,* vol. II. London: SCM Press.

Twersky, A. (1998) *Twersky on Spirituality.* New York: The Shaar Press.

van Deusen Hunsinger, D. (1995) 'Case study: Eva and her "black despairs".' In *Theology and Pastoral Counselling: A New Interdisciplinary Approach.* Grand Rapids: Eerdmans.

CHAPTER 13

Diversity in Care
The Islamic Approach

Faheem Mayet

Spiritual care

> The greatest disease in the West today is not TB or leprosy [or cancer], it is being unwanted, unloved and uncared for. We can cure physical diseases with medicine but the only cure for loneliness, despair and hopelessness is love. There are many in the world who are dying for a piece of bread but there are many more dying for a little love. The poverty of the West is a different kind of poverty – it is not only a poverty of loneliness but also of spirituality. There's a hunger for love as there is a hunger for God. (Vardey 1995, p.83)

Whenever people are confronted with terminal illness – which affects their very existence, threatening and changing their lifestyle or maybe even shattering it – then fundamental spiritual issues emerge. How this is understood by the NHS and the communities it serves is not the purpose of this chapter: that it has become an important aspect in the health of the physically fit and those who are ill is beyond doubt. The recovery of the patient within a known framework of religious belief adds immensely to his or her well-being when this support is offered during a stay in hospital and in the post-recovery period. Such a view is strongly supported by the growing literature about belief and health, evidenced by publications such as Sheikh and Gatrad's *Caring for Muslim Patients* (2000).

That Britain is now a plural society there is no doubt. We live, work and interact with people from diverse backgrounds, and most hospital populations comprise different people from a range of social and religious diversities. Various areas of our lives bring us into contact with people who have a completely different understanding of things we take for granted. This is especially true in the area of health care. A primary care development nurse mentions:

> Working in an area with a high ethnic population promotes many additional problems to those normally encountered in primary health care. Language barriers are the most obvious and unfortunately can mean that nurse consultations are not always as effective as we would like. Lack of understanding and education on the patient's behalf can cause problems with non-adherence to treatment, which can have a particular impact on diseases like diabetes and asthma. A lack of cultural awareness and understanding on the professionals' behalf can cause us to appear accidentally insensitive and thoughtless. (Hill 1999, p.296)

Most hospitals have come to terms with the fact that all patients, ethnic minorities included, should have access to spiritual care. But what spiritual care *is* needs definition. To the health care professional, spiritual care may simply mean that the hospital chaplain takes care of a patient, whilst faith groups may define spiritual care in a more specifically religious way. Islam, an all-encompassing faith, considers every facet of human life to fall in the domain of religion. Even simple aspects of daily life like sleeping, visiting the washroom, eating and dress are considered acts of worship when done in a manner prescribed by Islam. Spirituality is defined as the combination of the outer and inner aspect of actions of devotion, giving them their real significance. In a saying of the prophet Muhammad, peace be upon him, he is reported to have said: 'He who knows himself, knows his Lord.' This is clear reference to a level of self-awareness and understanding by humankind on the purpose of creation and meaning of life.

Thus with this view we are obliged to accept the fact that many patients will want answers to the issues facing them during their stay in hospital. A number of hospitals are now slowly beginning to recruit Muslim chaplains in their employment, allowing them an effective voice. Patients and staff consequently have access to a professional working with them in the delivery of 'quality care'. This is important because for many patients, their religious beliefs provide a framework within which to 'make sense' of things. Religious practices are a way of 'putting meanings to work' in the business of 'getting through' their illness (Simsen 1988, p.31). On a broader scale, speaking about the sociological aspects of religion, Dr Mohammed Omar Salem mentions:

Society can only survive if people share some common beliefs about right and wrong behaviour. Durkheim saw religion as a kind of social glue, binding society together and integrating individuals into it by encouraging them to accept basic social values. So, it is mainly through religion that an individual is socialized into the values of society. This set of moral beliefs and values may have been so deeply ingrained through socialization that it may have an effect on the everyday behaviour of believers and non-believers alike. (1999, p.47)

Islamic practice and terminology

Islam does not have an official clerical or theological body. There are no Muslim clergy and there is no hierarchy like that of the Christian Church. Islam invests the power of interpretation and decision making not in an institution but in the form of an expert. Experts are people proficient in Islamic law, who are of an upright and pious nature – the 'Alim' or Learned. In the past, most imams, ulama (scholars) and religious leaders acted in a personal capacity to provide help to patients in hospitals. The early Muslim doctor of medicine was trained as a religious scholar and acted as a religious adviser as well. Men like Razi, Ibn Sina, the Nestorian Hunayn Bin Ishaq and the Jewish scholar Maimonides were all scholars working in a clinical context. This brings us to the very term 'chaplain' and its inappropriate usage in the Muslim community. Many people will not be able to identify with the word. However, words like 'imam', 'moulana', 'shaykh' or 'mufti' are easily identified with Muslim professionals learned in their faith!

Hence, today, the very role of the 'chaplain' is brought into question. How can this term be used when any Muslim can in fact offer religious care? The giving of *spiritual* care, however, brings an added dimension to the realm of religion. The person giving spiritual care must not only be from a religious background but someone who is imaginative and understands the concepts involved in 'administering' care within a modern hospital organisation. In this way a Muslim scholar appointed by a Trust may not deliver religious care in the same manner as a Christian colleague. Supporting and enabling the relatives in giving such care, as well as acting as an intermediary between the community and the Trust, may form a substantial part of the work.

For example, a Christian colleague at another hospital was once surprised when asked to bring in a Muslim chaplain to attend to a very sick patient in intensive care. The Muslim chaplain spoke at length with the family but never went in to see the patient. This was because the family was fully capable of carrying out all the necessary religious and spiritual duties required. The role of the scholar was to advise the family about matters relating to the funeral – as well as to affirm and support them in their religious practice and faith at a critical time. This may not always be the case; obviously relatives may at times wish the scholar to spend time with the patient. Despite such variations in the way in which Muslim scholars work, for clarity within the organisation as well as a unity in the department, it is probably best for Muslim scholars to adopt the title 'Muslim Chaplain'.

The chaplain in the hospital

The work of all chaplains is in reality religious. It is now acknowledged that religion offers support and structures for coping with such stressful inevitable life events, such as:

- pregnancy, birth and child rearing
- marriage and divorce
- ageing and death.

In addition, the all-encompassing nature of Islam means that there are many aspects of a stay in hospital which may raise issues for the Muslim patient. For example:

- rituals related to worship, such as washing, prayer and fasting
- everyday customs, such as diet, dress and personal hygiene.

The next section of this chapter will discuss some of the life events and the Muslim customs associated with them, explaining their significance in the context of health care.

Life Events

Pregnancy and childbirth

Woven into the fabric of parenthood are a number of Muslim customs associated with this process. These include:

- The Adhaan: The five daily congregational prayers are preceded by a call to prayer, the Adhaan, which is said in Arabic throughout the Muslim world. The chaplain, father or elder member of the family will whisper this call into the right ear of the newborn child, whilst a similar call, the Iqaamah, is whispered in the left ear. It is greatly appreciated by the parents of the child if a private area or room is made available to the person officiating at this ceremony.

- The Tahneeq: Soon after birth and preferably before being fed, a small piece of date is softened then gently placed in the upper palate of the child. Again, a senior member of the family, the chaplain or imam at the local mosque usually performs this task.

- Circumcision: A requirement of Islamic law is that males should be circumcised as soon as possible. This has been a subject of much ethical debate, and chaplains can play a key role in advising their NHS Trust, as well as supporting the development of hospital-based procedures.

Child rearing

The most important aspect of spiritual and health care interacting is childbirth. The very process is itself a miracle. So much attention is paid to the newborn infant that the mother is now placed on a second level whilst the father is forgotten almost entirely! Yet, all three go through enormous physical and emotional changes from the onset. Questions are asked about the meaning of life and its continuity through children: what kind of future will the children face? Will we be good parents? The maternity clinic, with its busy schedule, will hardly have time for answering these serious spiritual questions.

One dimension of chaplaincy is therefore caring for patients going through the process of childbirth and how this affects them. For example, post-natal depression is an area where the second-level player has to be supported to overcome her state, by receiving proper care. It can be the case that in some Muslim families mental health needs are not well understood. In such a situation the work of the Muslim chaplain is to advise and support the family in the light of professional medical advice. This can involve the chaplain in speaking with the mother, father and wider family in order to encourage a better understanding of the illness and what its effects might be. Putting this into a religious context, the Muslim chaplain can emphasise that a woman suffering from post-natal depression deserves all the obligations of support due to any person who is unwell.

Handicapped and special needs children

This is an area that many chaplains may be ill-prepared to deal with. How do we comfort the couple, granted the gift of a child, albeit with a degree of deformity?

> When it comes to facing handicapped new life, and many have to do that, although there may be moral discussion as to whether that child should be allowed to live, or whether the mother should have an abortion, very little is done to discuss what the meaning of that life might be, what the value to society as a whole, to the family concerned, and to that child, of that life might be. Yet for many new parents facing that child, and the worrying about its future and their own wellbeing, it is those concerns, about meaning and hope, which are foremost in their minds. (Neuberger 1998, p.19)

In such a situation the Muslim chaplain emphasises the ethical principle that every child, no matter what their abilities, is a gift from Allah. A family might find this difficult to accept, and the chaplain therefore has a role in supporting them as they address their feelings towards their child and the changes he or she will bring to their life.

No children

A further dimension is the pastoral care of infertile couples. This is a challenge for chaplains from all faiths. How do we solve the ethical issues involved in some of the treatments that are on offer? In addition, there are spiritual issues to be coped with, as described by Rosemary Shaw:

> Infertility is *a crisis of identity*. What does it mean to be a man or woman? How do we communicate about painful topics? How do we make decisions? Intervention in the midst of this crisis can make the difference in a couple's capacity to function throughout their marriage. Also it is *a crisis of faith*. It makes one face one's own mortality. How does one cope with events outside one's control? How does one view God and Prayer? (1999, p.43)

Within all faiths such a situation may place enormous strains on a couple. It may be that they feel oppressed by the image of 'normality' generated by society or family expectations. A Muslim chaplain can offer help by emphasising the Qur'an's teaching concerning this; that while the bestowing of children is a blessing from Allah, the childless state is no less honourable. Many pious saints in Islam did not have children, but their contribution to their faith was in no way diminished. Helping parents come to terms with their position, and reconciling their feelings to their faith, can be an important task for a scholar working as a chaplain.

Marriage and divorce

Taking a view of health as a matter concerning the whole person, it is vital to consider wider factors in a person's life. Issues facing patients like an impending divorce or break-up of a relationship, custody of children, legal cost; the forthcoming wedding of a child or a relationship that needs to be defined within the parameters of religion, will certainly affect the religious and spiritual well-being of a patient. Thus how we relate these issues to the patient is vital for his or her well-being.

Ageing and death

Many religions have different teachings on how they wish their adherents to be treated in the face of imminent death. These will include how they wish to perform the last rites and arrangements for the patient's funeral. These details are important and can make a huge difference to the comfort of patients. The attendance of a chaplain can ensure that the hospital has a firmly placed policy on how to deal with the dying of patients within a particular tradition. The dying person in Islam should be permitted to leave this life in tranquillity. Ideally this should be in a familiar environment – preferably the home. The dying person should not be unduly disturbed, but accompanied in their last hours by the quiet prayer of their family. In the hospital it can be difficult to grant someone such an end, but the Muslim who works as a chaplain can do much to encourage the organisation to try and give the patient peace in their final hours. This is something for which all chaplains should work – no matter what their faith. Following death the expeditious removal of the body means much to the Muslim family. Again, the Muslim chaplain should do all that is possible to ensure that the hospital has appropriate procedures in place.

Worship, custom and ritual

Illness and a stay in hospital may result in anxiety for the observant Muslim patient. The two areas that can pose problems relate to worship and the particular customs that form part of the Muslim way of life.

Issues related to worship

Muslims pray five times a day, varying on the course of the sun in its rising and setting. Four principal postures are maintained in prayer, the standing, bowing, prostration and finally a sitting position. This can be difficult for patients recovering from illness. For example, a patient recently recovered from a hernia operation will no doubt ask the relevant questions about what postures are possible. Similarly, will the standing in prayer affect a patient who has had a major orthopaedic operation? Questions to be dealt with by the chaplain will include how to advise the patient who has limited mobility in performing the different postures of prayer, or is unable to move. The direction for prayer may also be an issue. Prayer should be directed towards Makkah and a patient may want his or her bed turned towards that direction.

Prayer is preceded by ritual washing of the hands, face, arms and feet. Again, there may be particular concerns for patients that the chaplain will need to attend to. A patient may want assistance with this or simply to know if they are excused from the task. There may also be questions of a more medical nature: will washing the face after a corneal transplant affect it?

The ninth month of the Muslim calendar, which is a lunar one, is called Ramadan. Muslims throughout the world fast from sunrise till sunset. A pre-dawn meal is taken to commence the fast and food is taken after sunset. Abstention from food, drink and sexual intimacy are necessary. The average fast, depending on the country, will be about 12 hours. In the UK, the winter months vary from 8 to 10 hours, from October to April; whilst the summer months will vary from 14 to 18 hours. Some patients may not be able to endure such a long length of time without food or medication. How will a patient come to terms with their seemingly weak expression of worship? This is where the chaplain will have to counsel patients and gently reassure them that Islam takes into consideration their physical state. For example, an insulin-dependent patient does not need food in quantity but, more specifically, needs the right foods at regular periods throughout the day. A Muslim scholar can encourage a patient with this illness that Allah requires a person to look after their body as much as to fulfil obligations of fasting. For a fast to harm the body would negate the spiritual benefits of fasting. It also possible for a patient to give 'fidyah' (compensation given for not being able to fast), which in turn is given to the poor. As with fasting, this almsgiving creates an identification with the poor, which is the purpose of the practice.

Religious festivals are an important consideration for Muslim patients and the relevant dates should be considered when making appointments for patients. The two major festivals, Eid ul Fitr, marking the end of Ramadan, the month of Ramadan itself, as well as Eid ul Adhaa, marking the Hajj (pilgrimage) and sacrifice, are times when Muslim patients would prefer not to come into hospital. The hospital's outpatient department would benefit greatly from the input of the chaplain in determining these times.

Everyday customs

Diet, dress and other personal issues are all seen within a religious context in Islam. For example, with respect to dress, many Muslims emulate or follow the Prophet Muhammad, peace be upon him, and his companions. Thus dress in Islam also has a very spiritual role. From the Eastern lands of Islam to the Atlantic, we find modesty and simplicity of dress that is emphasised in Muslim society. Tunics and sarongs for the people of Indonesia, Malaysia, Philippines and Bangladesh; changing to the loose shalwar kameez of India, Pakistan Afghanistan, Iran and Central Asia; the thawbs and kaftans of the Arab World and colourful gowns of Africa. Always emphasising looseness and simplicity in dress, discouraging exposure and immodesty:

> European dress is fundamentally out of keeping with the postures and gestures of Islamic worship; it hinders bows and prostrations, renders the prescribed ablutions more difficult, it takes away the dignity of the effortless sitting together on the flat ground; whoever wears European clothes is either a 'gentleman' or a mere worker or 'proletarian'. Whereas previously men were differentiated only by their culture, the community is all of a sudden split into economically determined classes and, with the cheap products of the factory, a poverty without beauty invades the home; ugly, senseless and comfortless poverty is the most widespread of all modern achievements. (Burckhardt 1992, p.162)

Islam's emphasis on simplicity means that clothing may be an important part of a person's spirituality. It also reflects beliefs about personal dignity and modesty. Such factors have their significance within a hospital and the Muslim chaplain may once again need to find a voice within the organisation to express this. The NHS's commitment to diversity raises as yet unanswered questions about the limitations of their policy. Is it, for example, acceptable for a Muslim midwife or other member of staff to wear 'purda' (facial veiling for women) whilst carrying out their duties? These are important discussions, and ones where a Muslim chaplain has a valuable role.

In terms of diet, pork is forbidden as is the meat of animals not slaughtered in the Islamic way, which is called 'halal' (permissible). Beef, lamb, camel, deer and chicken slaughtered in the Muslim way are accepted. Hospitals with Muslim patients need to consider the provision of halal food and avoid the contamination that can result from ill-trained and insensitive staff. Here, chaplains have a role in education for staff as well as – where appropriately qualified – authenticating sources of food supply. In order for any meal to be considered halal, it is necessary that the entire process from the raw source to consumption – preparation, cooking, freezing, storage and despatch – be strictly monitored and supervised by authorised Muslim personnel. If Islamic requirements are not followed, it would not only be incorrect and unethical but illegal to make any claim that this food is halal – even if such food bears the halal logo! (Institute of Islamic Jurisprudence 2000, p.A–7)

A further personal issue important to Muslims concerns physical contact between the opposite sexes. This is prohibited in most Muslim communities. Many Muslim women will prefer to see a female doctor or gynaecologist. Hand shaking also falls in this area of segregation and is something health care visitors should be aware of when visiting Muslim homes, followed closely by the rule of whether shoes should be removed or not. Also, what part of the home are they invited into, the male or female section of the house? For this reason Muslim chaplaincy within a hospital should only be begun on the basis that male and female chaplaincy staff are employed from the outset.

The road ahead

What can make chaplaincy even more effective? The question of what facilities are provided by a Trust for its chaplaincy department is vital. How does the inter-faith team work? At Dewsbury NHS Trust, the concepts of co-operation and belonging have been meaningful – members of the team are aware of where and when to ask for help and support in addressing issues. This has been the single most important factor for the successful development of multi-faith chaplaincy at the hospital. We trust each other and act as one body! If those faiths involved in chaplaincy share a common commitment to the care of the sick and their spiritual needs – in whatever tradition – then it is possible to develop strong bonds of common concern within a multi-faith team. Theological differences no doubt exist, but my experience is that they form points of intelligent discussion – not ideological dispute. A team that is imaginatively and ably led should be able to overcome and resolve what problems might exist – for example, in access to hospital information, the nature of facilities available and the future design of worship areas. It is not that there are no potential problems – it is whether or not the chaplaincy team is willing or able to address them in a constructive and mature way.

How can we prove we form a vital part in caring? An Associate Director of Nurses writing on the spiritual caring of patients aptly writes:

> Too often we work from the notion that hope is something the patient retains as long as sufficient information is withheld. When this is no longer tenable, we offer hope as a belief system that is 'delivered in propositional form', preferably by the chaplain. (Simsen 1988, p.33)

This obviously should not happen; rather both sides should realise the limitations of their roles and work together, as a team, to enhance the care that should be given. Both clinical and pastoral staff must realise this limitation of roles in supporting the patient. We cannot 'give hope' to another but we can support and encourage the hoping abilities of a patient. As chaplains, we can offer a caring relationship that permits rather than stifles the efforts of the patient to develop hope. We can stay with the person who is testing his or her own beliefs or struggling with questions of fear and faith (Simsen p.32). This is real caring, for those who listen day after day, exposing themselves to another's pain, are part of the healing process!

Finally, we have to ask ourselves, 'are we able to make a *real difference* to the patient?'

> The 16th century Spanish Mystic, John of the Cross, spoke about God as divine absence; and the way to God was the way of negation. Another analogy from the world of computers might help. Computers do not actually erase information when you delete a file, they simply lose the capacity to locate that information. It is somewhere in the system, but the computer no longer knows where. This is what the divine absence tries to express. God is there but no longer can be located because of the processes going on inside the person. (Sutherland 1997, p.16)

There is no doubt that those drawn into systems of health care often find the experience to be disorientating. For patients who find themselves in a religious or ethnic minority, that experience may be compounded. Attention to religious needs and practices can help such patients cope with their illness and the spiritual questions that it raises. Effective multi-faith chaplaincy also acts as a resource to the staff and organisation – raising the profile of spiritual issues in a unique way. By their presence in health care, chaplains help patients relocate God and in this we will be making a real difference!

References

Burckhardt, T. (1992) *Fez, City of Islam.* Cambridge: The Islamic Text Society.

Hill, S. (1999) 'A sensitive approach to issues of ethnicity.' *Practice Nurse 17,* 5.

Institute of Islamic Jurisprudence (2000) *The Institute of Islamic Jurisprudence UK Muslim Food Guide.* 3rd edn; Batley: Al Madinah Publication.

Neuberger, J. (1998) 'Spiritual care, health care: What's the difference?' In M. Cobb and V. Robshaw (eds) *The Spiritual Challenge of Health Care.* Edinburgh: Churchill Livingstone, 7–20.

Salem, M. O. (1999) 'Religion and psychiatry.' *Journal of Health Care Chaplaincy 2,* 14.

Shaw, R. (1999) 'Be fruitful and multiply.' *Journal of Health Care Chaplaincy 2,* 14.

Sheikh, A. and Gatrad A. R. (2000) *Caring for Muslim Patients.* Abingdon: Radcliffe Medical Press.

Simsen, B. (1988) 'Nursing the Spirit.' *Nursing Times 84,* 37.

Sutherland, M. (1997) 'Pastoral care, theology and mental health: relationship, discernment and wholeness.' *Contact 123.*

Vardey, L. (1995) *A Simple Path.* London: Ebury Books.

CHAPTER 14

No Level Playing Field

The Multi-Faith Context and its Challenges

Andy S. J. Lie

Professionals involved in health care readily acknowledge that anyone with a disease and illness is an individual with a wide range of needs. Patients are always more than just their bodies. Every individual has a name, a complex history and a personality formed out of a multi-cultural environment. The most appropriate health care is more than treatment of the physical symptoms and underlying pathology. For some people, the threat posed to them by disease and illness may increase their need for some form of religious activity. For many, however, any threat to their well-being will be met with a heightened sensitivity towards the search for deeper meaning and towards spiritual exploration and comfort. This perceived need will naturally impact on those who are close to that individual. What matters is not just cure or the lack of cure, but also the importance of healing (Aldridge 2000). These are naturally key concerns in a multi-faith society like Britain and, in particular, within the experience of both patients and staff in the NHS.

In this chapter, I shall draw upon my observations and experience of working in four hospitals (two acute, a women's and a children's) in Britain's second city, Birmingham. Inevitably, my position will be seen as somewhat ideological and context-specific, but it does not claim to constitute any definitive statement on the subject of multi-faith issues in health care.

Setting the scene

With the launch of the NHS in 1948, administrative frameworks and machinery were set in place to ensure the provision for the spiritual needs of patients and staff. A Christian chapel was usually set aside and each hospital appointed the number of chaplains it required. Appointments were almost entirely Church of England priests and were based roughly on the overall ratio of one full-time chaplain to 750 inpatients (Beckford and Gilliat 1996, p.21).

As time passed, this monopoly of the Church of England gradually gave way to ecumenical co-operation – that is, incorporating priests and ministers from the Roman Catholic and Free Churches (mainly Methodists, Baptists and the United Reformed Church). Nevertheless, the number of full-time Church of England chaplains grew from 183 to 266 in the seven years up to 1990 (Beckford and Gilliat 1996, p.21). Currently, of approximately 350 full-time chaplains in the UK, only 35 are Free Church and 15 Roman Catholic (Booth 2000, p.18), the corollary being that chaplaincy managers or team leaders are still predominantly Anglican.

It is within this context that the changing needs of patients in British society must be considered. It is now estimated that about ten per cent (5.75 million) of the population have community backgrounds outside Britain (Parekh 2000b, p.372). Ethnic and religious diversity is now a fact of British life. Necessarily, it is also a fact of life for the NHS. On the one hand, the number of managers, senior managers and senior clinical staff in the NHS nowhere reflects the wider demographic reality; on the other, minority ethnic staff are somewhat over-represented at the lower levels of the health service (Parekh 2000b, pp.188–189). In some major British cities, the number of patients from the minority ethnic and world faith communities in the hospitals can be extremely high. Multi-ethnic and multi-faith Birmingham, with its approximately one million population, is an obvious example.

Whither official guidelines?

The Patient's Charter (DoH 1991) set out the standards of service a patient can expect to receive in primary and secondary care. Privacy, dignity and religious and cultural beliefs are to be respected 'at all times and in all places'. That last phrase is absolutely telling as it can put an enormous pressure on staff at the coalface of service delivery. Soon after, in 1992, the NHS Management Executive issued important Health Service Guidelines on 'Meeting the spiritual needs of patients and staff'. This document is still the official and primary basis for NHS Trusts in terms of recommending religious and spiritual provision. The guidelines were essentially meant for health service management to decide how to provide for the spiritual needs of patients and staff, based on consultation with those who can provide such services, and how to co-ordinate such provision. The carefully drafted guidelines were purportedly multi-faith and made no favourable preferences for Christians.

In 1996, seminal research was produced by Beckford and Gilliat as part of 'The Church of England and Other Faiths' project. The work contained the following important findings:

- Essentially, both in civic religion and in publicly funded chaplaincies (namely, prisons and health care organisations), the Church of England/Anglican clergy remained the primary gatekeepers. Their status and influence had, in fact, been augmented by the NHS reorganisation of the 1990s with members of other faiths (and in some instances, members of other Christian churches) still relying on Anglicans to provide access to facilities and resources.

- Although members of the world faith communities were neighbours alongside Christians, without the equal opportunity to participate in publicly funded religious activities, political empowerment seemed an ever-distant prospect.

- Despite the Church of England's facilitation of the limited access for other faiths, mounting pressures on resources in health care organisations made it increasingly difficult for Anglican chaplains to treat all faith communities in an even-handed fashion.

- Hence the challenge for the future. In view of the above factors, and especially the fact that the world faith communities in Britain are large enough and established now, can they assert their independence from Anglican patronage or oversight?

Also published in 1996 was the NAHAT document *Spiritual Care in the NHS: A guide for purchasers and providers.* This significant publication built upon *The Patient's Charter* and the twin values of equity and quality, pointing to the very few good practices already in existence and proposing an expanded spiritual, religious and cultural care department for hospitals to adopt. These two pieces of work from the mid-1990s remain highly relevant for the year 2000 and beyond. The situation in many NHS hospitals has progressed little towards a more inclusive approach. Church of England territoriality (with all its vestiges of power and authority) is still a force to be reckoned with in British public life, despite the fact that the actual number of people attending Anglican churches today just about hovers above the one million mark. At the time of writing, new and long awaited guidance is due to be issued to the NHS through the Multi-Faith Joint National Consultation process, headed up by the Hospital Chaplaincies Council. However, any sea-change in spiritual care provision will require courage and the mustering of will among senior managers and policy makers. Official directives by themselves will not achieve this.

Multi-faith chaplaincy: is that possible?

While many in the NHS would like to see things moving faster in the direction of equity, the fact is that for the foreseeable future, religious and spiritual care will continue under the domain of Christian chaplaincies. In any acute NHS Trust, the bulk of chaplaincy sessions remains Christian, usually shared among the major denominations, with at best very few paid sessions, if any, allocated to one or two other world faiths. Be that as it may, there have been some rays of hope in some hospitals. In Birmingham, sessional Muslim chaplains have been appointed since the late 1990s at the psychiatric, children's, women's and university hospitals. In the university hospital there is a very limited amount of money allocated for Hindu, Sikh and Jewish advisers as the numbers for these three faiths are far less than that for Muslims. The pressing need then is for more resources to be committed to employing chaplains from all the world faith communities. One innovative suggestion put forward by a Birmingham community leader is to appoint a full-time chaplain of a world faith (for example, from the Hindu communities) who could work across the main hospitals, each with a small percentage of staff and patients from that particular faith. Besides overcoming the logistical difficulties and co-ordinating the financial machinery, this approach has the potential of drawing together the various chaplaincies and hospitals in a creative partnership.

As volunteers have traditionally played a role within the Christian chaplaincy service, we are now beginning to see some individuals from other world faith communities serving as volunteers in hospitals. However, the services of volunteers should not be relied upon to meet the needs of patients from minority faith communities as an alternative to paid staff. This can result in exploitative situations whereby minority faith leaders provide a service for free which should be paid for by the chaplaincy. Examples of this have been documented recently: an imam was found to have provided sessional input to a major London hospital on a regular basis without payment for nine years (Orchard 2000, p.60).

It is not uncommon these days to note the claim (for example, through advertisements for job vacancies) that a certain department is 'multi-faith'. However, it is far from clear how many purportedly multi-faith departments have paid staff on their books. Many have at best one or two sessional staff from the faith communities (mainly Muslim), while remaining predominantly Christian. Others are likely merely to hold a list of contacts of local faith communities and their religious leaders whom they can call on for help only in times of urgency. Hence, the implication is clear. It is very difficult for the sessional (for example, Muslim) chaplain's views to be heard at higher levels of the organisation, let alone for them to have any sort of co-ordinating role. Responsibility for major decisions will continue to lie with the Christian chaplaincy manager, who is most likely to be Anglican.

What appropriate terms may we use?

An issue which is likely to raise much discussion in multi-faith chaplaincies is that of terminology. Up to now, I have used the term 'chaplain' or 'chaplaincy' quite loosely. These terms have their Christian roots and fairly universal usage, and over the years have been borrowed increasingly by other world faiths. Are there more neutral terms like 'spiritual care' and 'spiritual care givers' or 'religious advisers' which could be meaningfully used? If a different term, for example 'imam', is used, what status will that Muslim person have alongside the Christian chaplain in the ward? The fact is, as things are at present, most if not all patients and staff are so used to the term 'chaplain' that other terms will find it difficult to catch on in common vocabulary. Yet, if the essentially Christian term 'chaplain' is used for everyone, does it not compromise the distinctiveness of each of the other faiths? If different terms are used for different faiths, then only those with 'chaplain' titles (especially if they are Christian priests or ordained ministers) will be acknowledged and others could be relegated to a second-class or third-class existence. Furthermore, instead of calling it the 'chaplaincy', is there a much more viable and acceptable term for a spiritual care department that could be developed for use in the 21st century?

Religious and spiritual needs: how do we define them?

In any multi-faith society, therefore, it is crucial that other models of spiritual care are sought, moving away from the traditional focus of the Christian priestly mode offering 'pastoral care', where the term itself connotes a strong Judeo-Christian bias. This raises two further questions. First, how do we resist the pressure to mould other world faiths according to the Christian model? Second, are circumstances conducive enough so that new models of spiritual care could evolve naturally? Who and what, then, should we look for when hospital managers recruit and retain members of other world faiths to complement the work of the Christian chaplains? Is it always necessary to have the theologically trained or religiously qualified person? Should we not actively seek other creative possibilities – the social worker, link worker, counsellor, teacher, community specialist, health care professional – each with a deeply held religious faith and practice? How do we assess the suitability of these potential candidates when they do come forward? Will they have some kind of organisational support for the spiritual care that they will undertake? I am not just referring to the staff support within the hospital, but also to support in the community. These are pertinent questions to consider, especially if there is a strong council of faiths present in a city that could support their members when they undertake important religious and spiritual duties (both paid and voluntary) in hospitals.

Sacred space

The provision and further development of 'sacred space' in the current NHS hospital settings are fraught with thorny issues. Christian chapels, be they in the form of a Victorian chapel guarded by inflexible rules, or a modern user-friendly adaptable room, will be available for use in most hospitals. The question is: if they could, how should they be altered and adapted for multi-faith use, assuming that other spaces are not available? If other rooms are available, which faith groups should gain access to this extra space? If the full renovation costs are not borne by the hospital authorities, should the users look to the various faith communities for help? If Muslims are supposedly the next largest faith group represented among staff and patients in many situations, should there be a Christian chapel, a Muslim prayer room and a third space for the others? What is beginning to develop in NHS hospitals is the certain provision of the Christian chapel, while all other faiths can use a small designated 'multi-faith' room. This suggests that 'multi-faith' does not include Christians at all. Whereas in the earlier discussion on chaplaincy, 'multi-faith' predominantly means a Christian department with some very loosely attached personnel from other world faiths, 'multi-faith' in sacred space could mean anything other than Christian. This apparent shift in definition is quite remarkable, especially when the users themselves are often not aware of it.

In any case, what makes a space 'sacred' is also a question worth asking. What is almost certain is that in any multi-faith contexts, it behoves the planners and policy makers to make provisions of space that rightly reflect not only the area's demographic reality but more importantly, its potential and actual clientele. At the time of writing, there are plans to incorporate an imaginatively designed multi-faith centre for a new university hospital planned for Birmingham in 2007.

Practical challenges: data and training

Most hospitals face basic difficulties in gathering accurate figures on the number of patients from the various world religions and of no specific religious affiliation. The figures below give the religious composition of patients in an acute Trust in Birmingham in 1998:

Faith	Average % of patients
Buddhist	0.04
Christian	56.53
Hindu	0.96
Jewish	0.31
Muslim	3.98
Sikh	1.04
Others	0.63
None	2.94
Not given	33.57

The figures show that one of the main problems is patients not providing information on their religious affiliation. There may be many reasons for this: some may genuinely not know, some may not have been asked and others may simply refuse to divulge the information. There is a further complication to the collection of accurate statistics. As the current record system stands, there are possibly more than 20 different Christian denominations alongside single entities like Buddhist, Hindu, Jewish, Muslim and Sikh. If one religious group (that is, Christian) is accorded heterogeneity, that feature should be recognised in other world faiths. Some records do not even register Baha'i or Jain.

A further practical challenge concerns the need for the education and training of all staff towards cultural competence in service delivery. However, before we attain cultural competence, steps have to be taken in terms of cultural awareness training, the building up of cultural knowledge and the developing of cultural skills. These features of cultural competence must also be supported by real-life cultural encounters (Campina-Bacote 1994). There is now a fast-growing field and a large corpus of literature and expertise built up around the subjects of ethnicity and health care, transcultural care, language and interpreting issues and inter-cultural communication (Henley and Schott 1999).

Training in these fields is absolutely indispensable for all staff, be they in the front line of clinical care or in policy making. Yet it is important to realise that within the time constraints, lack of resources and work pressures which staff face in the health service, these training programmes are at best generic in nature. Staff, if they have undergone basic training in these fields, will need to adapt their understanding of issues to their local areas of work. The inherent danger in any such schemes of training is the unwitting by-product of crude stereotypes – the 'reification of the culture of minority ethnic groups as static, monolithic entities that can be categorised by an index of stereotypic cultural traits' (Lambert and Sevak 1996, p.155). In its crudest form, at the ward level, imagine a staff nurse encountering a Hindu, a Muslim and a Sikh, and thinking they should all have *halal* meals because they come from a South-Asian background. Developing culturally competent service delivery demands that health care professionals be fully aware of the complex interplay of influences that constitute 'culture' and the detailed empirical knowledge that should undergird their practice.

Concluding remarks

Throughout this chapter, the absence of a level playing field has been evident. I now wish to conclude with the following reflections.

First, we return to an earlier question: can we ever move away from Church of England patronage and oversight? If that is not possible in British civic life, can it be realised in the health service? Will NHS senior management have the moral will to challenge current Anglican superiority in institutional spiritual care?

Second, bearing in mind that chaplains of world faiths other than Christian are a comparatively recent phenomenon in the health service, how do we prevent their distinctive *modus operandi* from being absorbed into the wider ocean of the traditional approaches of Christian chaplaincy? Here, I have in mind the tendency among many Christian chaplains to engage in *generic* chaplaincy. The dangers of this approach have been identified as a confusion of professional roles with resulting inadequate spiritual care (Engelhardt Jr. 1998).

Third, we encounter social justice concerns in the sense that not only is there inequality in access to health care, but there is no equitable distribution of human talents and skills in the health service either (Parekh 2000b, pp.176–191). The physical and other needs are there, but they are not always appropriately met by the right kind of personnel. Bhikhu Parekh is correct in reminding us that 'equal rights do not mean identical rights' in a multi-cultural society (Parekh 2000a, pp.239–263).

Fourth, the corollary then is that the twin fault lines of religious discrimination and institutional racism must be acknowledged. This is specially relevant in view of extending the legislation on religious discrimination (currently investigated by the British Home Office and the University of Derby) and the coming into effect of the Human Rights Act in October 2000, followed by the Race Relations (Amendment) Act in April 2001. What the future augurs only time will tell. But surely the challenge is to aim towards multi-cultural Britain as 'a community of citizens and a community of communities' (Parekh 2000b, p.ix).

Fifth, some of the issues discussed above impinge on ethics in terms of the problems of resource allocation. Experience shows that if there is an available empty space in a corner of a hospital, the likelihood is greater that it will be used as a clinical area or for the purpose of generating income rather than a place of prayer. Not for a moment do I pretend that capital and service planning are easy matters, but the example attests to the fact that the 'unseen' aspects of health care are often relegated to the bottom of priorities.

Last but not least, there is a dearth of writings on the subject of religion and health care in the multi-faith context. Material on spiritual care emanating from Christian perspectives is widespread and it is remarkable that, for example, a most recent article by Booth (2000) hardly mentions the multi-faith reality within the NHS. However, things are slowly changing with the appearance of Clarke (1998), Markham (1998) and Lewis (1999). Notwithstanding these recent developments, a key question remains: how do we move beyond *ex cathedra*-style pronouncements on multi-faith issues in health care into more meaningful and fruitful discussions, which are grounded in the realities of service provision and supported by empirical inquiry?

Acknowledgement

The main substance of this essay was first presented as The Roger Hooker Memorial Lecture 2000 to a joint meeting of the Birmingham Council of Faiths and the Council of Christians and Jews (Birmingham branch). I am deeply grateful to The Revd Stephen Barton, Chaplaincy Manager at Birmingham Women's Hospital, for his very helpful and constructive comments on earlier drafts of this essay.

References

Aldridge, D. (2000) *Spirituality, Healing and Medicine: Return to the Silence.* London: Jessica Kingsley Publishers.

Beckford, J. A. and Gilliat, S. (1996) *The Church of England and Other Faiths in a Multi-Faith Society.* Warwick Working Papers in Sociology. Coventry: University of Warwick.

Booth, H. (2000) 'Spiritual care in the National Health Service.' *Epworth Review 27,* 4, 13–21.

Campina-Bacote, J. (1994) 'Transcultural psychiatric nursing: diagnostic and treatment issues.' *Journal of Psychosocial Nursing 32,* 8, 41–46.

Clarke, R. (1998) 'Report of the Multi-Faith Joint National Consultation between all Spiritual Care Givers and Hospital/Health Care Chaplaincy Organisations working within the NHS, 20–21 October 1997.' Unpublished paper of the Hospital Chaplaincies Council.

Department of Health (1991) *The Patient's Charter and You.* London: HMSO.

Engelhardt Jr., H. T. (1998) (issue ed) 'Generic chaplaincy: providing spiritual care in a post-Christian age.' *Christian Bioethics 4,* 3, 231–315.

Henley, A. and Schott, J. (1999) *Culture, Religion and Patient Care in a Multi-Ethnic Society: A Handbook for Professionals.* London: Age Concern England.

Lambert, H. and Sevak, L. (1996) 'Is "cultural difference" a useful concept? Perceptions of health and the sources of ill health among Londoners of South Asian origin.' In D. Kelleher and S. Hillier (eds) *Researching Cultural Differences in Health.* London: Routledge.

Lewis, C. (1999) 'Religion and spiritual care.' *Theology CII,* 809, 336–344.

Markham, I. (1998) 'Spirituality and the world faiths.' In M. Cobb and V. Robshaw (eds) *The Spiritual Challenge of Health Care.* Edinburgh: Churchill Livingstone.

NAHAT (1996) *Spiritual Care in the NHS: A Guide for Purchasers and Providers.* Birmingham: National Association of Health Authorities and Trusts.

NHS Management Executive (1992) 'Meeting the spiritual needs of patients and staff: Good practice guidance.' London: Department of Health.

Orchard, H. (2000) *Hospital Chaplaincy: Modern, Dependable?* Sheffield: Sheffield Academic Press.

Parekh, B (2000a) *Rethinking Multiculturalism: Cultural Diversity and Political Theory.* London: Macmillan.

Parekh, B (chair) (2000b) *The Future of Multi-Ethnic Britain* (The Parekh Report). London: Profile Books.

Contributors

Rabbi Martin van den Bergh is Senior Hospital Chaplain of the Visitation Committee of the United Synagogue, Rabbi of Wembley United Synagogue and holder of the Welfare Portfolio on the Chief Rabbi's Cabinet.

The Very Revd Dr Wesley Carr is Dean of Westminster. He has served in Chelmsford Cathedral and as Dean of Bristol. He also has a long association with The Tavistock Institute of Human Relations.

Revd Mark Cobb is Senior Chaplain at Sheffield Teaching Hospitals NHS Trust, an Honorary Lecturer in the Faculty of Medicine at the University of Sheffield and an Honorary Research Associate of Lincoln Theological Institute, University of Sheffield.

Dr Sophie Gilliat-Ray is a Research Fellow in the Department of Religious and Theological Studies at Cardiff University.

Revd Martin Kerry is Senior Chaplain at Nottingham City Hospital NHS Trust.

Andy Lie is Multi-Faith Facilitator at University Hospital Birmingham NHS Trust and Birmingham Women's and Children's Hospitals.

Revd Dr David Lyall is Principal of New College and Senior Lecturer in Christian Ethics and Practical Theology at the University of Edinburgh.

Mufti Faheem Mayet is Senior Muslim Chaplain at Dewsbury Health Care NHS Trust and Co-ordinator of the Madrassah for the Mount Pleasant Islamic Trust, Batley.

Wilfred McSherry is Lecturer in Acute Care of the Adult at the University of Hull.

Dr Helen Orchard is Honorary Research Fellow at Lincoln Theological Institute, University of Sheffield and an ordinand at Westcott House, Cambridge.

Stephen Pattison is Head of the Department of Religious and Theological Studies at Cardiff University.

Revd Christopher Swift is Trust Chaplain at Dewsbury Health Care NHS Trust and a research student at Lincoln Theological Institute, University of Sheffield.

Revd Dr Margaret Whipp is Consultant in Palliative Medicine at St Benedict's Hospice, Sunderland and Director of Academic Development for the North East Oecumenical Course.

Revd Dr James Woodward is Master of the Foundation of Lady Katherine Leveson, Director of the Leveson Centre for the Study of Spirituality, Ageing and Social Policy and the Bishop's Adviser for Health and Social Care in the Diocese of Birmingham.

Subject Index

Name Index